12/2/15
$18.00

Dosed

The Medication Generation Grows Up

KAITLIN BELL BARNETT

Beacon Press
Boston

Beacon Press
25 Beacon Street
Boston, Massachusetts 02108-2892
www.beacon.org

Beacon Press books
are published under the auspices of
the Unitarian Universalist Association of Congregations.

15 14 13 12   8 7 6 5 4 3 2 1

This book is printed on acid-free paper that meets the uncoated paper
ANSI/NISO specifications for permanence as revised in 1992.

Text design and composition by
Wilsted & Taylor Publishing Services

Many names and identifying characteristics of people mentioned
in this work have been changed to protect their identities.

Library of Congress Cataloging-in-Publication Data
Bell Barnett, Kaitlin, 1983–
Dosed : the medication generation grows up / Kaitlin Bell Barnett.
p. ; cm.
Includes bibliographical references.
ISBN 978-0-8070-0134-9 (hardback : alk. paper)
I. Title.
[DNLM: 1. Mental Disorders—drug therapy.
2. Adolescent. 3. Child. 4. Mentally Ill Persons—psychology.
5. Psychotropic Drugs—adverse effects. WM 402]
616.89'180835—dc23   2011037253

To my parents,

who taught me to love stories

Contents

Introduction

I fall hard for coming-of-age stories, and my list of favorite books and movies contains many in this genre, from *Pride and Prejudice* to *The Catcher in the Rye*. The movie *Garden State*, which starred Zach Braff and Natalie Portman, also struck a chord with me when it came out in 2004. It dramatizes a few days in the life of Andrew Largeman, a twenty-six-year-old struggling actor in Los Angeles who returns to his native New Jersey for his mother's funeral. Andrew is nothing if not alienated: he feels disconnected from celebrity-studded Hollywood as well as from his old hometown, which he hasn't visited since leaving for boarding school nearly a decade earlier. For the first time in sixteen years, Andrew has stopped taking the psychotropic medications his psychiatrist father prescribed after ten-year-old Andrew caused an accident that rendered his mother a paraplegic. Like the illegal drugs his high school buddies take, Andrew's meds serve as a metaphor for the feelings of inadequacy, disappointment, and rootlessness endemic to my generation of twenty-somethings. Judging from the film's cult-hit success, its target audience of my peers apparently found the metaphor apt. When Andrew falls in love with a quirky, vibrant girl he meets in a doctor's waiting room, she shows him how to reengage with his feelings—and the world. Presumably, he leaves the medications behind.

For several years, *Garden State* remained my favorite movie about my generation. It spoke to me as a young person growing up in turn-of-the-millennium America—though not as a young *medicated* person. In fact, I completely forgot psychiatric drugs were even mentioned. Funny, because I myself have been taking medication since high school, and *Garden State* is one of just a couple of films I know of to allude to the psychological impact of growing up taking psychotropic drugs. But although it touches on this important phenomenon, the film never really examines its underlying assumptions that medications numbed Andrew's pain and guilt, and that getting off them allows him once again to experience the agony and ecstasy of life.

For the first time in history, millions of young Americans are in a position not unlike Andrew's: they have grown up taking psychotropic medications that have shaped their experiences and relationships, their emotions and personalities, and, perhaps most fundamentally, their very sense of themselves. In *Listening to Prozac*, psychiatrist Peter Kramer's best-selling meditation on the drug's wide-ranging impact on personality, Kramer said that "medication rewrites history."[1] He was referring to the way people interpret their personal histories once they have begun medication; what they thought was set in stone was now open to reevaluation. What, then, is medication's effect on young people, for whom there is much less history to rewrite? Kramer published his book in 1993, at a time of feverish—and, I think, somewhat excessive—excitement about Prozac and the other selective serotonin reuptake inhibitor antidepressants, or SSRIs, that quickly followed on its heels and were heralded as revolutionary treatments for a variety of psychiatric problems. For most people, I suspect, medications are perhaps less like a total rewriting of the past than a palimpsest. They reshape some of one's interpretations about oneself and one's life but allow traces of experience and markers of identity to remain. The earlier in life the drugs are begun, the fewer and fainter those traces and markers are likely to be. All told, the psychopharmacological revolution of the last quarter century has had a vast impact on the lives and outlook of my generation—the first generation to grow up taking psychotropic medications. It is therefore vital for us to look at how medication has changed what it feels like to grow up and to become an adult.

• • •

Our society is not used to thinking about the fact that so many young people have already spent their formative years on pharmaceutical treatment for mental illness. Rather, we focus on the here-and-now, wringing our hands about "overmedicated kids." We debate whether doctors, parents, and teachers rely too heavily on meds to pacify or normalize or manage the ordinary trials of childhood and adolescence. Often, the debate has a socioeconomic dimension that attributes over-medication either to the striving middle and upper-middle classes, or to the social mechanisms used to control poor children and foster children. We question the effectiveness and safety of treating our youth with these drugs, most of which have not been tested extensively in children and are not government-approved for people under eighteen. We worry about what the drugs will do to developing brains and bodies, both in the short and long term. The omnipresent subtext to all this: what does the widespread "drugging" of minors say about our society and our values? Certainly, these questions are worth debating—even agonizing over. But they ought not to constitute the be-all and end-all of our society's conversation about young people and psychiatric drugs, particularly with millions of medicated teens transitioning into adulthood. Too much of the discussion occurs in the abstract, and drugs too easily become a metaphor, as in *Garden State*, for a variety of modern society's perceived ills: the fast pace of life and the breakdown of close social and family ties; a heavy emphasis on particular kinds of academic and professional achievement; a growing intolerance and impatience with discomfort of any sort. Far too rarely, though, do we consult young people themselves. How do *they* feel about taking medication? How do *they* think it has shaped their attitudes, their sense of themselves, their academic and career paths, their lives? How do they envision medication affecting their futures?

Focusing on people who needed therapeutic intervention early in life and who continued to use medication for an extended period of time can help us get past the are-they-or-aren't-they nature of the "overmedicated kids" debate. By assessing what medication has actually meant for my peers, I hope to get at something more intimate and more complex than either the psychotropic true believers or the total skeptics allow themselves to consider. "A prescription becomes an event that generates fantasies, wishes, concerns, and meaning," write the social scientists Tally Moses and Stuart Kirk in an analysis of young people's experiences of psychotropic meds. "It structures one's own expectations and those of others in ways that are not necessarily intended or foreseen."[2] As Moses and Kirk suggest, the experience of taking psychotropic drugs is more than just popping a pill, and these drugs often become a part of the self in ways children and teenagers could not have imagined when they swallowed their first dose. Now that the first generation of medicated kids is entering adulthood, we have an invaluable opportunity to hear about their experiences with psychotropic drugs, and their assessment of those experiences. In addition to looking at the family, medical, and educational circumstances in which drugs are prescribed and taken, that is what this book sets out to do.

My cohort lives with some powerful contradictions. On the one hand, we have grown up with the idea that prolonged sadness, attention problems, obsessions and compulsions, and even shyness are brain diseases that can—and ought—to be treated with medication, just as a bodily disease like diabetes ought to be treated with insulin. The 1990s, sometimes called "the Decade of the Brain," encompassed a period of unprecedented growth in understanding how the brain works, which generated enormous enthusiasm about the prospects for discovering the underlying mechanisms behind mental illness, enthusiasm that many say was overwrought and premature. Direct-to-consumer pharmaceutical advertising on TV, which the U.S. Food and Drug Administration authorized in 1997, has allowed drug companies to define the public's understanding of mental illness and psychiatric medications—and this is especially true, I think, for young people who knew no other paradigm. Even as we grew up, though, immersed in the idea of an "imbalance" of particular brain chemicals—an outdated theory that has not held up to the science—we have inherited the American ideal of self-sufficiency, of solving one's problems through one's own resourcefulness. As we've sought to forge our identities, we have often struggled to reconcile the two.

· · ·

It took me a while to conceive of my medicated peers as a coherent group, much less one deserving of a book-length study. Until recently, I would not even have included myself in the category of people whose formative years were shaped by psychotropic drugs, let alone shaped in any profound way. When I began taking Prozac at age seventeen, I didn't spend a lot of time contemplating whether I'd lose some essential aspect of my identity, and I certainly didn't consider myself a part of any larger societal phenomenon. I was only vaguely aware that various drugs like Prozac had become available in the late 1980s and through the 1990s, and that they had helped a lot of people.

Before taking Prozac, I had spent two years in therapy with first one therapist and then another. To a depressed adolescent, two years feels as though it's an eon. I thought it was time to give medication a try. I was far less concerned with the implications of taking a psychiatric drug than I was with banishing the exhausting and oppressive symptoms of my pervasive unhappiness: the apathy and hopelessness, the irritability and boredom, the pessimism and incessant self-criticism. For several years these symptoms had seemed to colonize my entire being, and when they abated after a couple of months of Prozac, I credited the medication. I figured a "chemical imbalance" must be to blame, and skipped the philosophizing. Even when Prozac seemed to stop working five years later and I began, in desperation, trying a battery of other antidepressants and antianxiety drugs, I still basically swallowed the pills and left it at that. The drugs only mattered to me insofar as they treated, or failed to treat, my symptoms.

Then, shortly before my twenty-fifth birthday, seven years into my life on medication, I read a column in the *New York Times* about a young woman in her early thirties who had been taking antidepressants almost continuously since she was fourteen. Richard A. Friedman, the young woman's psychiatrist and a frequent contributor to the science section of the *Times*, noted that the patient "credited the medication with saving her life." But, he wrote, she had also begun to struggle with the "equally fundamental question" of how the drugs had shaped her psychological development and, ultimately, her identity. Noting the huge increase in the number of youths taking antidepressants and other psychotropic drugs, Friedman postulated that his patient was just one of innumerable people entering adulthood with such concerns. With little scientific data on how drugs affect the developing body and mind, he added, these were problems for which few answers were forthcoming.[3]

I was intrigued. Since I didn't relate to the woman's doubts and anxieties, I wondered whether starting medication at a younger age than I did, at a more vulnerable and unstable period in her emotional development, had contributed to her discomfort. I can't say the article suddenly prompted me to start questioning who I'd be had I never taken Prozac, but it did make me intensely curious about my peers. *Who are these people,* I wondered, *and why are they so ambivalent about their medication?* I didn't know anyone who fit the bill, so I began looking.

I talked to friends of friends, current college students and recent graduates I met through campus mental health groups, and I joined online forums for mood and behavior disorders, both those devoted specifically to psychotropic medication and more general sites where people post their medical data and histories, such as PatientsLikeMe. Since I identified myself as a journalist, I suspect most people didn't want to talk to me at all, fearing public disclosure of a private, online identity. Others shared my initial, uncomplicated assessment: the medication worked, therefore, they must have had a biochemical malfunction in their brains, as much a disease as diabetes and no more profound.

The more stories I heard, though, the more it seemed that even people who believed, on balance, that the drugs helped them—somehow made them more stable, motivated, focused, reliable, or upbeat—still entertained plenty of ambivalence about issues such as what side effects the medications caused and how to understand their identity while taking a drug that affected their mood, behavior, and maybe even their entire personality. Some harbored these suspicions from the get-go; others developed them over time. "At first, I thought, 'Oh, okay, yeah, that'll make me feel better,'" one young woman from outside Boston told me of her experience beginning antidepressants at age eleven. "And then it entered my consciousness more that it was something more serious . . . that had stronger effects on my being."

Although qualms and questions exist among people of all ages who take psychiatric meds, the more I talked with young adults, the more I came to realize that many of the queries and worries were directly linked to and intensified by the process of coming of age. The same large themes kept appearing. In what ways, and to what extent, had psychotropic drugs shaped them into the people they had become? How had their problems and symptoms shifted over time, and what role had the meds played in those shifts? Did they still need medication, or might they have outgrown their old problems? They speculated about the implications of being diagnosed and treated for a chronic disease at an age when they were supposed to be models of health. They puzzled about how taking a prescription drug had affected their body image, their sexuality, their attitudes toward alcohol and other mind-altering substances, and their sense of their own abilities to control their emotions and behaviors. One young man whom I met online put it bluntly. "The areas that have most been affected by my medication use. Huh. All of them." A twenty-one-year-old woman who had been taking stimulants and antidepressants since age eight explained plaintively, "I always had this idea of figuring out who I am—and not who the medication makes me."

My interviewees' questions and answers struck me as more compelling than I had expected, but I was still pretty sure that I didn't have much in common with them. The writer Andrew Solomon has said that depression is "the aloneness within us made manifest,"[4] and I would add that for many this isolation includes the unshakable conviction that you are uniquely miserable, that no one shares or could possibly grasp the complexity of your wretchedness and the plight that desolation causes. I have certainly felt that way when I was depressed; neither Prozac nor any of the other drugs I've taken convinced me of the banality of my distress. As far as I was concerned, I had been uniquely unhappy—not necessarily unhappier than other people, but unhappy in a way particular to me. The miracle of medication for me was that it had erased my despair without making me feel stripped of myself.

Later, after a lot of reading and interviewing and researching, I realized my melancholy was hardly unique. But you might forgive me for having believed it was, as I didn't discuss my medication use with anyone except my immediate family and some close friends—and even then, only in passing. What was there to discuss, now that the symptoms I suffered as a teenager had more or less disappeared? I'd experienced some side effects and even some alarming new symptoms, but how could medication—the solution to my problems—pose any kind of fundamental dilemma? Very few people, for that matter, had discussed their own medications with me. If the subject came up, it was in the abstract, a snide remark that a friend or acquaintance "*really* should be medicated," or in some vaguely moralizing debate over whether stimulants such as Adderall and Ritalin gave some of our peers an unfair academic edge, or whether learning disabilities had been misdiagnosed as attention deficit hyperactivity disorder (ADHD) and might be better treated through other means. Yes, there were other people my age taking medication, but I certainly didn't feel any sort of cheesy, self-help-group connection to them.

Even as I began talking to people in my basic situation, I remained skeptical. How could their experiences have any meaningful commonalities one could extrapolate to larger truths? To be sure, these people were all "medicated," but they had been diagnosed with vastly different conditions, and they were taking a large array of very different types of psychotropic drugs. Several of them (echoing experts in the mental health field) cautioned me against lumping everyone together. Taking a short-acting stimulant like Ritalin, they said, was vastly different from taking a long-acting antidepressant like Prozac, which, in turn, was totally different from taking a mood stabilizer like Depakote, or a powerful atypical antipsychotic like Zyprexa.

Having been trained both as a journalist and a historian, though, I harbored a conviction that people, myself included, were products not only of their individual experience but also of their culture and their era. There was no denying that my peers and I had lived through—had indeed been the vanguard of—the psychopharmacological revolution. Prozac was not the first of the selective serotonin reuptake inhibitor antidepressants, but it was the first to hit the U.S. market, gaining

FDA approval at the end of 1987. Thanks to national education campaigns trumpeting depression as a major public health issue and a period when, due to changes in FDA requirements, few new psychiatric drugs were introduced, Prozac made a huge splash.[5] Other SSRIs such as Zoloft and Paxil followed a few years later. Starting in the early 1990s, new kinds of antipsychotic medications were released. Originally used for schizophrenia, these "atypical antipsychotics" were increasingly prescribed to stabilize the mood swings of childhood bipolar disorder and to quell irritability associated with autism and behavior disorders. Longer-acting formulations of the stimulant Ritalin, which had been used in children since the 1950s, appeared, as did other drugs for attention deficit/hyperactivity disorder. By the mid-1990s, the prescribing of psychotropic drugs to children was front-page news in major newspapers. When I entered college in 2001, college counseling centers were reporting an overwhelming influx of patients, including growing numbers who arrived at school with a long history of mental illness and medication.

Since reliable statistical analyses lag years behind actual shifts in medical practice, the statistics about the actual number of kids prescribed medication began to hit the media when these children had already entered adolescence, or even adulthood. When the data did emerge, it confirmed what people already sensed, a massive increase in the number and percentage of children being treated with psychiatric drugs. Although children and teenagers were—and still are—prescribed such drugs less frequently than adults (with the exception of stimulants), the rate of growth is remarkable. Between 1987 and 1996, the percentage of people under twenty taking at least one such drug tripled, from about 2 percent of the youth population to 6 percent,[6] at minimum an increase of more than a million children. Between 1994 and 2001, the percentage of visits to doctors in which psychotropics were prescribed to teenagers more than doubled: to one in ten visits by teenage boys and one in fifteen visits by teenage girls between the ages of fourteen and eighteen.[7] In 2009, 25 percent of college students were taking psychotropic meds, up from 20 percent in 2003, 17 percent in 2000, and just 9 percent in 1994.[8] The prescribing of more than one medication has become far more common in child psychiatric patients in recent decades—even though, as the National Institute of Mental Health's head of child and adolescent psychiatry research noted in 2005, there was "little empirical evidence of efficacy and safety from well-designed studies."[9] Although statistics about medication use show a clear increase, nationally representative data is still severely lacking.

Many children and teenagers were also facing the prospect of taking medication for far longer than people who first encountered psychotropic drugs in adulthood. In the 1980s and 1990s, doctors tended to prescribe drugs for a limited period of time for both adults and children, except for bipolar disorder and schizophrenia, long considered intractable, lifelong conditions. But it became increasingly clear to doctors that ADHD persisted into adulthood in about two-thirds of people, and that an early bout of anxiety or depression often portended more frequent and more severe episodes later in life. And so my peers and I found that a drug initially prescribed by a pediatrician as a stopgap measure for some alleged hormonal or developmental problem often became a long-term, perhaps indefinite commitment.

The medical profession wasn't the only force driving the increase in prescriptions. Our parents, the ubiquitous baby boomers, are notorious for seeking medical solutions to every ailment (one book on the subject, by journalist Greg Critser, cheekily dubbed them "Generation Rx"). The boomers also tend to be portrayed as overly indulgent parents, obsessing endlessly about their children's fragile self-esteem and all-important academic performance. They wanted us, their children, to be not just happy, fulfilled, and confident, but also high achievers from a young age. They worried that their children could come under the influence of—or be outright harmed by—the unhappy, disaffected kids who captured headlines in the 1990s for their dramatic suicides or school shoot-outs. The boomers tried to be cooler or more hip than their own parents, but most of them were far from "anything goes" when it came to their offspring. As one of my subjects put it, describing his parents' and teachers' expectations, "You can't not function. You can't wake up in the morning and not be able to function." The goal, he said, was to strike a magical balance between being "happy-go-lucky" and "efficient." These conflicting expectations and aspirations produced some rather stressed-out children—and some parents, teachers, and doctors readily inclined toward pills to help manage the effects of that stress.

My peers and I also came of age in a time when the economics of health insurance were changing drastically. In the 1980s and 1990s, most employer-based health insurance moved toward a managed-care model, and state- and federally funded health coverage for children expanded. The government and the HMOs were both eager to keep costs down, and therefore preferred relatively cheap psychiatric drugs to long-term talk therapy (despite a growing medical consensus that the most effective treatment for most psychiatric conditions was a combination of medication and therapy).

Meanwhile, a shortage of child psychiatrists, especially in poor and rural areas, meant that many troubled children could not see a specialist. As a result, already-busy pediatricians shouldered more of the burden of treatment: in the late 1970s, about 7 percent of all visits to pediatricians involved a child with emotional or behavioral problems, but by the mid-1990s, that rate had nearly tripled.[10] Increasingly, those visits involved writing a prescription. Prescribing data collected between 1992 and 1996 showed that pediatricians prescribed 85 percent of psychotropic medications.[11] As psychiatrists switched from forty-five-minute visits with time for psychotherapy to fifteen-minute "med checks," prescriptions often came with little continuing discussion about how kids felt about taking medication, or how it was affecting them. That was fine by some, but not by others. One young woman I interviewed, who received her prescriptions from time-crunched psychiatrists who scheduled fifteen-minute appointments they often cut short, wished there had been time to "talk about feelings, not just symptoms." One young man told me that even though psychiatric medication is "so much a part of our culture," he could "probably count on one hand" the conversations he'd had about his medication use, or anyone else's.

Most psychotropic drugs, it's important to note, were and still are prescribed to children and teens without official FDA approval for the relevant condition and age group. As long as clinical trials have shown a given medication to be safe and, under certain narrow requirements, effective for some condition, and as long as the pharmaceutical companies don't advertise a drug for a nonapproved use in kids, doctors can legally prescribe it "off-label." Off-label prescribing to children is nothing new, in large part because concerns about the ethics and legality of conducting drug trials on minors have plagued medical research for decades. (As the pediatrician and pharmacologist Henry Shirkey observed in a 1968 article in the *Journal of Pediatrics*, children were becoming "the therapeutic orphans of our expanding pharmacopoeia," and people calling for drugs to be tested in children were still reiterating Shirkey's formulation three decades later.)[12] Historically cautious, doctors used to wait a number of years after a new medication came on the market before prescribing it to children. But with all the hoopla surrounding the introduction of new psychotropic drugs in the late 1980s and 1990s and an influx of young patients seeking treatment, fewer doctors bothered to wait.

This sharp increase in prescribing made the lack of research all the more acute. Controversies brewed. Did antipsychotic drugs cause dangerous obesity and early-onset diabetes? Did stimulants stunt growth or increase the risk of drug abuse later in life? Did taking antidepressants or stimulants before puberty predispose children to bipolar disorder in adulthood? Did SSRIs like Prozac increase the risk of a teenager attempting suicide?

In the late 1990s, responding to the precipitous rise in prescribing and what researchers called a shameful lack of safety and efficacy data, the National Institute of Mental Health began funding a series of major, multisite medication trials in children and teenagers. They led to some important findings, with trials for major depressive disorder and obsessive-compulsive disorder concluding, for example, that combined medication and cognitive-behavioral therapy (CBT), a short-term therapeutic treatment focused on refocusing thought and behavior patterns, was the optimal regimen for the greatest number of children, compared to a placebo or to either medication or CBT alone.[13] These so-called "multimodal" studies were groundbreaking because they were some of the first to compare the efficacy of different treatments, measuring one drug against another, drugs against therapy, and standardized, carefully managed treatment against "community care," the treatment a child would ordinarily receive in his or her local area. They also were comparatively long-lasting, which produced certain notable findings. For example, children in the government's major ADHD trial at first seemed to do best on medication alone, compared to various other combinations of treatments. But when the same children were assessed two years after the study ended, there were no differences in either ADHD symptom reduction, or improved school or family relationship functioning, among different treatment groups. Medication's superior effects, in other words, did not last.[14] The vast majority of studies are not this wide-ranging or long-term. As a result, myriad issues remain unsettled and hotly debated today and continue to bedevil parents, doctors, and young people as they weigh the relative risks and benefits of embarking on psychopharmaceutical treatment.

Recently, some studies have questioned the efficacy of antidepressants for mild and moderate depression in adults, which has generated considerable public interest and raised questions in many people's minds about the wisdom of taking the drugs at all, let alone long term.[15] In fact, as psychiatrist Peter Kramer pointed out in a column in the *New York Times*, this particular new evidence only applies to episodic, not chronic and chronically recurring, depression, and it doesn't say anything about the drugs' efficacy for many other conditions, including numerous anxiety disorders, severe depression, menstrual-related mood disorder, and the depressive phase of bipolar disorder.[16] Other studies have raised troubling questions about how some psychotropics may affect the brain long term; the drugs are effective at preventing relapse for as long as they are continued, but some evidence suggests, for example, that the changes the drugs cause may set patients up for withdrawal symptoms that look very much like relapses, prompting, some have argued, a kind of psychological dependence on the drugs.[17] The studies have generated considerable controversy in the mental health profession and in the popular media.

Overall, extended, decades-long longitudinal studies tracking outcomes of medication treatment in kids remain close to nonexistent, because of the great expense and effort involved in tracking people over many years. As a result, the original group of medicated children has entered adulthood with very little information about the lasting physical, emotional, and cognitive effects of using psychiatric medication during childhood and beyond. They are left with the legacies of using medication, though in many cases they're not quite sure what those legacies are, or will be.

I don't mean to suggest that every young adult who spent his child or adolescent years taking medications is preoccupied with the existential implications of that treatment. Undoubtedly, many would contend, as some of my interviewees initially did, that the effects were simple: the drug either worked to resolve symptoms, or it didn't. But I suspect that, as was the case for many people I interviewed, taking a little time to reflect on a drug's role in their own coming-of-age stories would allow them to see just how wide-ranging and complicated the impact of medication has been. Thus, this book focuses on exploring the legacies of medication, while placing them in a larger cultural and sociological context. I have tried to provide a basic, clear assessment of what's known, from a scientific and medical perspective—as well as what remains unknown—about how psychiatric drugs affect the developing brain, body, and psyche. To that end, I have interviewed medical and social science researchers, as well as clinicians who have counseled young adult patients who have been taking drugs since childhood. My thinking has been informed by historical accounts, memoirs, and academic studies from many fields, along with newspaper and magazine articles about psychopharmacology and childhood mental illness from the past three decades. A small group of social scientists has begun studying the subjective or "lived" experience of medication use in young people. Their research, and that of sociologists and medical anthropologists interested in people's experience of illness and treatment, has shaped my thinking. But the backbone of this book consists of the individual stories of my peers, the people whose voices have been drowned out amidst the clamor of researchers, doctors, politicians, school administrators, and, yes, parents.

No book can encompass the totality of a generation's experience, and I don't pretend mine will be able to do that for psychiatric medication and mental illness. I do hope that it provides an instructive range of perspectives and experiences. Since I have aimed for depth over breadth, I have chosen to focus on a few people who represent a variety of medical conditions, geographic locales, and socioeconomic backgrounds, supplementing their perspectives with those of others I interviewed. Examining young people with long histories of psychiatric medication has to some extent skewed my focus toward more seemingly intractable mental problems. In part, this is because more serious mental illnesses tend to be diagnosed earlier; in part because the people whose experience with medication is more fraught are those who have the most to say and who wanted to talk for this book. I found most of my subjects through social media groups and chat rooms dedicated to medical and psychiatric issues, groups that are admittedly more likely to attract people still struggling to treat their disorders, though certainly a large number of them live full, productive, and successful lives. As many of them have observed, the drugs help keep them from bottoming out, but they don't make everything perfect. "When you get into this issue of having people take these medications for a long period of time, at some point you have to ask, 'What is the goal of the treatment?'" one of my interviewees asked. Is erasing the symptoms the goal, he wondered, or learning how to cope with them? What is the definition of "recovery?" "Because, as you probably know," he added wryly, "no psychiatrist will ever tell you you've been cured of depression or anxiety. You're only in remission."

I have found considerable variation in people's experiences and assessments of their medication and its impact on their development. Some people have stuck with one or two drugs over many years; others have cycled through multiple diagnoses trying virtually every drug available. Some have formed intimate relationships with their therapists and psychiatrists; most have had their treatment limited to "med checks" with psychopharmacologists. Some people's parents pushed hard for medication; others opposed it strongly. Some credit medication with saving their lives; some think it ruined portions of their lives. Just as striking are a single person's shifting views and relationships to medication over time. The drugs influence one's life story, of course, but experiences and circumstances, so much in flux as one comes of age, also influence how one perceives and thinks about the drugs.

As a result, interviews with my subjects about events that happened to them ten, fifteen, or twenty years ago are necessarily colored by what they have learned and experienced since then, although I have tried as much as possible to distinguish what they knew or felt at the time from what they realized or decided later. I have tried to present my subjects as three-dimensional characters, not as medical patients whose treatment exists in a vacuum. Consequently, I discuss the forces, individual, familial, and societal, that led them to take medications and explore how the experience of taking these drugs substantially affects their lives. To some extent I take my subjects at their word since my goal is to understand how they feel about taking medications, but I also try to step back and analyze the broader implications of their experiences. Clearly, my own perspective is influenced by the fact I am writing about my peers—as well as the fact that I have been taking various medications for anxiety and depression for over a decade. I have referenced my own experience or point of view when I thought it would add to the narrative, or when I felt it shaped my analysis of larger trends or other people's accounts.

Taking psychotropic drugs is an individual, sometimes lonely, act. Many have criticized it as an individual, piecemeal solution to larger societal problems better solved through collective action. For young people accustomed to near-constant digital connectivity and to sharing the most intimate personal details online, taking medication is a bit of an anomaly, a peculiarly solitary experience (I'm struck, for example, by how few young people blog about their medication, though, admittedly, it's hard to measure the frequency of Facebook or Twitter updates). This is not a self-help book, but it does offer some new ways of thinking about what it means to take medication from a young age. Almost all of the people who agreed to be profiled in depth for this book said they did so because they thought it was important to help others understand what it's like to be young and medicated. They want to inform not only their peers, but also their parents' and grandparents' generations, as well as young children and teens, and the parents of those kids, who are considering embarking on drug treatment, or who want to know what the experience is like and what may lie ahead. And they want to encourage others to speak out about growing up on medication, a topic much discussed by others but far too rarely discussed by the young people who have lived through it.

CHAPTER I

Difficult Kids

Difficult kids suffer and cause much suffering
to parents, sibs, teachers, and other kids.
Everyone feels great and understandable pressure to do something.

—ALLEN FRANCES, TASK FORCE CHAIRMAN,
Diagnostic and Statistical Manual
of Mental Disorders-IV

Claire, age eleven
HUDSON, OHIO / 1991

In the summer of 1991, Claire Frese was eleven years old and felt she had the weight of the world on her shoulders. After days spent swimming with friends in the lake across the street from her big, white house, she lay awake at night, staring at a collage of magazine cutouts that covered one entire wall of her bedroom. She had made it expressly for the purpose of distracting herself from the thoughts that filled her head while the rest of the family slept peacefully. Sometimes, she thought listlessly about the utter pointlessness of life, about how you spend your whole life working, just trying to make a living, and then you die. Other times, she lay awake gripped with worry—about war, about world hunger, about her own destruction. In her journal, where in happier times she wrote about the crushes she had on boys, or about fights with her girlfriends, she envisioned instead elaborate, dark scenes of her own rape and murder.

Until this summer, Claire's parents had seen her meltdowns, her sleeping troubles, and her worrying simply as aspects of her personality. Compared to her brother, Joe, two years older, and sister Bridget, eighteen months younger, Claire seemed always to have been an extraordinarily sensitive child—a difficult child, in her more trying moments. From birth, she had cried often and slept poorly. As a blond, round-eyed, fat-cheeked toddler and preschooler, she was bright, alert, and talkative but wildly averse to certain sensations, like the texture of particular foods, or the feeling of a brush running through her hair. For as long as she could remember, she had had little mantras she repeated to quiet herself, especially when she was nervous: "I'm scared and I wanna go home" was one, even when she was safe in her own bed.

In grade school, she was exquisitely and painfully attuned to teasing from her peers and had spent part of third grade at home, so poorly did she react to bullying from a former friend. Never one to keep her emotions to herself, she cried when teased, and when provoked or frustrated at home was subject to dramatic meltdowns; if she was unhappy, she was taking everyone down with her. Usually, her parents had little patience for the outbursts. They either sent her to her room or just ignored her and walked away.

To a large extent, Claire's sensitivities seemed to her parents to be simply part of who she *was*—and she was also warm, loving, and deeply empathetic. This assumption was shaped by the thinking on child development current in the 1980s, when an increasing emphasis on children's inborn characteristics replaced the parenting dogma of nurture and upbringing that had dominated the middle decades of the twentieth century. Recent child development research, including groundbreaking experiments by the Harvard developmental psychologist Jerome Kagan, had shown that almost from birth different children experienced and reacted to the world in very different ways, and that to some extent these differences in temperament persisted well into adolescence and even adulthood.

Even if these traits were just part of who Claire was, though, she and her parents couldn't help but notice that her moods and behaviors became dramatically more volatile the summer before she was to begin middle school. At first, her mother, Penny, chalked up Claire's worsening moods to lack of sleep and preteen hormonal changes. She and Claire's father, Fred, decided to see how Claire fared when she began middle school in the fall. Bright and highly motivated to achieve, she loved school.

But when Claire began sixth grade, she spiraled rapidly, breaking down in tears in class and at home over homework and forgotten books and assignments. The school administrators maintained that Claire was no more moody or dysfunctional than many of her schoolmates, but the Freses didn't consider her meltdowns to be ordinary preadolescent behavior even for a "sensitive" child like Claire. Claire had always been something of an attention seeker and prone to histrionics. Still, they had read enough to know that when a child threatens suicide, even obliquely, saying things about life not being worth living, or just wanting to end it, one needs to take her seriously. They booked an appointment with her pediatrician, seeking some kind of explanation for her behavior and, they hoped, treatment.

The pediatrician gave Claire a full physical exam and told the Freses something that hadn't occurred to them. He thought Claire was probably depressed. He referred the Freses to a therapist. And he did something else, too, something that was quite unusual for the time. He prescribed Claire an antidepressant.

The year was 1991. Until very recently, the options for treating a disturbed child were limited, drastic, and expensive. In previous decades, children with crushing developmental disabilities would have been institutionalized, though the 1970s and 1980s saw a move to integrate both children and adults into the community and keep them living with their families. Children with a history of trauma, those with severe behavior problems, phobias, separation anxiety from parents, or serious problems adjusting to a new sibling, a new school, or a new town, for example, might see a psychologist, family therapist, or behavioral therapist if their parents had the money or sufficient insurance coverage, although by the mid-1970s insurance companies were cutting back on reimbursements for long-term therapy, citing insufficient evidence of effectiveness (although evaluating effectiveness was complicated by the fact that there were literally hundreds of techniques).[1] Conducting therapy with children, moreover, could be difficult and time-consuming for myriad reasons, not least the difficulty of distinguishing normal processes of development from pathology and the challenge of wooing an often-recalcitrant child, who typically did not choose treatment, to open up to a stranger. This last point of who initiates treatment is important, according to author and child psychiatrist Kevin Kalikow, since "the child might not have the insight to understand the problem as a problem or the perspective to be able to look at him or herself from the outside." Play therapy and role-playing, which sought to uncover some of the child's internal or unexpressed conflicts, could yield quite telling results, but these techniques required considerable patience and skill on the part of the therapist.[2]

In the eleven years since Claire's birth, in 1980, a lot had changed in the world of mental health in general, and in children's mental health in particular. Invigorated and excited by an explosion of new psycho-pharmaceuticals beginning in the 1950s, psychiatry had largely moved toward a "medical model" of mental illness that increasingly explained pathology as the result of chemical dysfunction in the brain rather than psychological reactions to traumatic events, a shift the pioneering child psychiatrist Leon Eisenberg summed up in 1986 as going from "mindlessness" to "brainlessness."[3] Reflecting this change, in 1980 the American Psychiatric Association published a radically revised manual for diagnosing psychiatric problems. Previous editions of *The Diagnostic and Statistical Manual of Mental Disorders* (*DSM*), which first came out in 1952, were heavily influenced by Freudian thought, which viewed neuroses as the result of inner psychological conflicts stemming from one's experiences, primarily in childhood. The 1980 version of the manual, in an effort to demonstrate that the profession could diagnose illnesses consistently and reliably, not simply based on a single psychiatrist's opinion, was purged of Freudian influences and embraced instead a new "descriptive psychiatry," classifying different disorders based on lists of symptoms divorced from the patient's external circumstances. The American Psychiatric Association launched a massive public relations effort to hype the manual and, as former *New England Journal of*

Medicine editor in chief Marcia Angell has described it, the *DSM* came into "nearly universal use, not only by psychiatrists, but by insurance companies, hospitals, courts, prisons, schools, researchers, government agencies, and the rest of the medical profession."[4] The manual included rating scales that categorized various traumatic disruptions (the birth of a new sibling, for example, or the death of a parent), but explicitly did not make these psychosocial considerations necessary for a diagnosis. The result was that a child could receive a diagnosis of mental disorder independent from what was happening in her life.

When it was released in 1980, the *DSM-III* allowed for children to be diagnosed with adult mental illnesses, such as depression, schizophrenia, and obsessive-compulsive disorder, although it also introduced a category of disorders that were "usually first evident in infancy, childhood or adolescence."[5] Longitudinal studies following people for many years, as well as retrospective studies based on interviewing adults with psychiatric disorders about their pasts, showed that a very high percentage had started experiencing symptoms in childhood or adolescence. (Recent data has borne out these reports, indicating that half of all lifetime cases begin before age fourteen and three-fourths before age twenty-four.)[6]

By the early 1990s, when Claire was diagnosed, doctors also had more incentives to treat children with emotional or behavioral disorders. Studies showing elevated rates of drug abuse, crime, and other troubles in adults and teenagers with untreated ADHD suggested that early intervention might help, though some researchers worried that treating children with stimulants might make them more prone to substance abuse later in life. The risks of untreated depression were also becoming clearer, as longitudinal studies indicated that depression and bipolar disorder had a cumulative effect, with each depressive or manic episode putting the sufferer at risk for more frequent—and more serious—episodes down the road. If mental illness could be stopped early in its tracks, the thinking went, perhaps children could be inoculated against later suffering.

Many baby boomer parents of the 1980s and '90s were drawn to this new biological paradigm of mental illness in part because it potentially cast them as partners in their child's treatment, rather than as a source of their neuroses, as the previous Freudian model had done. In past decades, analysts had blamed cold "refrigerator mothers" for childhood autism and adult schizophrenia, and indulgent mothers for little boys' hyperactivity and disruptive behavior. Certainly, by the final decades of the twentieth century plenty of psychotherapists and analysts took a more nuanced view of the parent-child relationship and worked hard to enlist the parents' help in altering children's behaviors. Psychoanalyst and child development expert Stanley Greenspan blended the two schools of thought, titling the first chapter of his popular 1995 book, *The Challenging Child*, "You're Not the Cause, but You Can Be the Solution."[7] Greenspan's philosophy acknowledged the roles of both "nature" and "nurture" in children's problems, but to many parents, simply being told that their child had a "biological disorder" sounded comparatively appealing.

Thus, by the 1990s, doctors and parents who were so inclined not only had something to call troubled children besides "difficult" or "sensitive"; they also had reason to begin treatment early in the hopes of staving off a worse course of illness. Perhaps most importantly, beginning in the 1990s, doctors also had new tools at their disposal for treating these problems, as a rash of new psychiatric medications, ushered in by Prozac's blockbuster success, began to hit the market. The number of psychiatric medications for anxiety, depression, and psychotic disorders had been proliferating since the 1950s, but the only class of drugs with an established track record in young people had been stimulants, primarily Ritalin and, to a lesser extent, Adderall, Dexedrine, and Cylert, all of which had been on the market for years and were used in children for treating attention and hyperactivity problems. Most of the other psychotropics were considered either ineffective or unsafe for kids.

During the 1980s, however, one class of drugs, the tricyclic antidepressants, named after a chemical structure that includes three rings of atoms, showed some promising results in children for treating a range of issues, including bed-wetting, severe childhood phobias, attention deficit/hyperactivity disorder (ADHD), and depression. Accordingly, what limited data exists shows that tricyclic prescriptions to children increased between two- and threefold from 1988 to 1994. In 1991, the year Claire's pediatrician diagnosed her with depression, about five in every one thousand kids aged two to nineteen and enrolled in managed care insurance, as opposed to Medicaid, took a tricyclic antidepressant, most commonly as a second-line treatment for ADHD after they didn't respond to stimulants.[8] At the same visit in which Claire's pediatrician diagnosed her with depression, he prescribed one of these tricyclics.

Despite some initial enthusiasm about their use with depressed children, tricyclics turned out not to work very well; studies in the late 1980s and early 1990s found no significant difference between depressed children who took a tricyclic and those who took a placebo. The tricyclics weren't ideal from a safety perspective, either. In high doses, they could be toxic, even fatal. In 1980, the Associated Press and other news outlets reported a Food and Drug Administration campaign to alert parents about the drugs' dangers, citing statistics that a thousand children under age five were sent to emergency rooms each year after accidentally swallowing the drugs; five hundred had to be hospitalized, and ten died.[9] Even in therapeutic doses, tricyclics were known to increase heart rate and blood pressure in children; in fact, a year or two before Claire received her prescription, medical journals had reported the sudden unexplained deaths of three children who had been taking the tricyclic desipramine for ADHD. Later in the decade, several more such deaths were reported.[10] Some doctors began to worry about whether the medications were worth the collective risks.

Claire's pediatrician didn't discuss any of those risks with the Freses, but they had a sense he was not in favor of giving adult medications to children and that he considered the medication a short-term, emergency measure, until they could get Claire into therapy. They were just relieved that he had been prescient enough to recognize Claire's troubles as depression. Compared to the average parent in 1991, Fred and Penny Frese were probably far better situated to spot mental illness in their children. For fifteen years, Fred, a psychologist who had himself been diagnosed with paranoid schizophrenia at age twenty-five, was director of psychology at the state's largest adult psychiatric ward. Yet they hadn't been able to identify Claire's problem. Because of the family history, they knew that Claire and her siblings were at increased risk of mental illness; they simply hadn't expected anything to show up so early. Nor had Claire exhibited many of the classic signs of adult depression, such as acting withdrawn, mopey, or uninterested in the things that she usually enjoyed. And despite her anxious insomnia, she'd spent the summer swimming and playing with her friends. Only later did they learn that psychiatrists had recently come to recognize extreme irritability as a major symptom of depression in children and adolescents.

The idea that Claire could be depressed because of an organic problem in her brain, rather than because of trauma, neglect, or other difficult experiences, made perfect sense to the Freses. In the decade following his diagnosis in his mid-twenties, Fred had been hospitalized ten times, and he had endured therapists who tried to delve into his past for what they suspected were the traumatic roots of his illness.[11] With medications, however, he had been able to lead a successful life as the head psychologist at Ohio's largest inpatient psychiatric unit, a father of four, and, later, an advocate for people with schizophrenia. Claire knew her father had a mental illness and that except for the occasional brief relapse he functioned very well. She also knew he was himself a psychologist. However, she seemed to have somehow picked up certain negative associations with either therapy or mental illness in general. Before her first appointment, she wrote her mother a journal entry saying she was scared to go to the session, lest the therapist decide she was "crazy."

The first therapist they consulted acted like a television caricature, limiting his involvement to scribbling notes and saying "Um hmmm" and "Tell me more about that." The second one spent the first several sessions plumbing for indications of abuse or neglect. When he couldn't find any, he told the Freses that Claire was one of the best-adjusted children he'd encountered in all his years of practice. It couldn't have helped that Claire assiduously avoided any discussion of her moods or behavior. At first, afraid of being deemed "crazy," she had pretended to see only cheery images in the inkblot tests (she eventually admitted she'd been fudging her answers, and the psychologist redid the test). Later, when she decided the psychologist didn't think she was crazy after all, she took advantage of the sessions as an opportunity to gossip about kids in school. She'd always been a chatty kid, and she was thrilled that for an hour every week or so, she had a captive audience. In the car on the way home, she'd provide Penny with replays of the sessions. Inevitably, she would have avoided any mention of her dark moods, her poor school performance, her suicide threats, or anything else that was causing trouble at home. Penny would say, "Didn't you tell him about how your medications aren't working?" or "Did you mention that you threw all those glasses the other day?" and Claire would say, "Of course not! I don't want to talk about that."

Penny told the psychologist she didn't think Claire was telling him the whole story and that he ought to talk with her and Fred, too. He seemed irked that they were telling him how to do his job and responded with a few perfunctory phone calls. "Okay. Go ahead," he'd say. "What do you have to tell me?" In the meantime, he continued to dig for signs of abuse or drugs. When Claire told him she knew what he was looking for, but that she'd experienced no such thing, he said, "Well, that's what your mother would like you to think." That was the last time the Freses saw him. They gave up on therapy and pinned their hopes on Claire's medication.

Everyone enters medication treatment with some kind of expectation, conscious or unconscious. Indeed, part of what drove the increase in the prescribing of psychiatric medications during the 1990s, especially the new selective serotonin reuptake inhibitor (SSRI) antidepressants, was the widely hyped promise of a miracle transformation. I was one such person; I went into my antidepressant treatment at age seventeen disillusioned with therapy and holding out great hope that Prozac would rescue me. Publicly, I didn't gush about the wonders of the medication— I was almost a little embarrassed that my stubborn misery had been felled so quickly by a little pill—but privately, I considered myself a changed person, reunited with the "real me" I'd felt alienated from since puberty.

A skeptic might call this the placebo effect, but not all of people's suppositions about medication are positive. Nor do expectations exist in a vacuum. We all bring culturally influenced attitudes to our medication treatment. But young people in particular are influenced by the beliefs and behaviors of the important adults around them—their parents, their teachers, and their doctors.

So what kind of expectations did a child like Claire have in the early 1990s, when psychotropic drugs in general, not to mention psychotropic drugs prescribed to children, played a much smaller role in our cultural consciousness? It's probably fair to say that most children's awareness of mental illness, not to mention their awareness of the drugs increasingly used to treat it, was extremely limited—at least until later in the decade, when, in a significant move, the FDA allowed pharmaceutical companies to begin advertising directly to consumers on television.

Claire didn't know of any other children in her school taking psychiatric medication, but she had grown up in a household where psychopharmaceuticals were both a part of her father's work and part of the family routine. Claire couldn't remember her parents explicitly using the word "schizophrenia" until she was about nine, but they had made it clear to her and her siblings that Fred took medication for his "nervous problems," just as he took heart medication. When her older sister, her dad's daughter from his first marriage, was prescribed Prozac at college about a year before Claire got her antidepressant prescription, Penny and Fred explained that to the kids, too.

So Claire didn't find the idea of taking medication to tweak troubling emotions and behaviors threatening or foreign. If her mom and dad and the doctor wanted to call her feeling of separateness "depression," fine. And if they had a medicine that would treat it, she'd go along, just as she'd go along if her mother or father told her to take penicillin for an infection, or Tylenol for a fever. She trusted them. It didn't occur to her to worry about any risks.

Clearly, not all children begin medication so willingly. The fact is that they don't have to consent to treatment; their parents or caregivers do. Their initial desire for medication and their reaction to it depend, not surprisingly, on the nature of their relationship with those caregivers, and whether and to what extent they understand the medication's purpose. Growing up in Fort Lauderdale, a little boy named Paul received his medication for the first time under far from ideal circumstances. The trauma associated with this introduction would shape his attitude about his treatment for years to come.

Paul, age five
FORT LAUDERDALE, FLORIDA / 1993

In the parenting books of the 1980s and 1990s, a "difficult child" wasn't just a discipline problem; he was, as the child psychiatrist David Fassler put it succinctly in a parent-guide chapter title, "everybody's crisis"— a threat to the entire family dynamic that needed to be addressed and dealt with.[12] Increasingly, the resolution to the crisis involved psychiatric medication.

This view assumed that the family was functioning well before the child started having problems. Clearly, plenty of families weren't, although the calmly reassuring tone of the parenting books, aimed at a middle-class audience of educated, attentive parents, didn't often acknowledge this. Paul came from the kind of family that was more likely to inspire government reports or sober newspaper editorials than parenting guides. Yet, over the course of several years, in more foster and group home placements than he could count, and after endless monitoring by caseworkers, psychiatrists, psychologists, and teachers, Paul would come to think that he, not his unstable and traumatic upbringing, was the problem. He would also come to hope, for a time anyway, that medication might fix him.

Until he was five, Paul lived with his mother and three sisters in a poor section of Fort Lauderdale just off the interstate. Like many in the neighborhood, his parents were both immigrants, among the waves of refugees fleeing the brutal political repression and devastating poverty that troubled Haiti during the 1970s and '80s. His father never seemed to have a steady job; his mother worked in a series of fast-food restaurants. They lived separately in adjacent apartment buildings and had a stormy, often violent relationship. Oftentimes, Paul's sister, who was just three years older, was left in charge of Paul and their two baby sisters. His mother, who was partially disabled and walked with a severe limp, had trouble keeping tabs on Paul even when she was home. Often, he just ran out the door, knowing that because she was handicapped, she wouldn't be able to chase him down. From time to time, his father showed up at their apartment in a rage and beat up Paul and his mother. Paul was never sure if his parents loved him or not.

Rival gangs composed of African Americans, Jamaicans, Hispanics, and Haitians populated the neighborhood. Roaming the streets with his friends, Paul developed an ethic of toughness, learning from a very young age to fend off attacks and to assert himself. At school, he was energetic and talkative, but often disruptive. Teachers suspected something was wrong at home—he was absent from school almost as much as he was there. When he came to school one day covered in bad cuts and bruises, someone called child welfare. On that occasion, the bruises came from older kids in a rival gang, not Paul's dad. In any case, when child welfare officials arrived, they determined that the house, run down and infested with pests, seemed safe for his three sisters, but not for five-year-old Paul, since his mother couldn't keep him from running off into the street at night. They placed him in a hospital.

At first, the hospital seemed to Paul like a magical haven from the violence of both his home and his neighborhood. He swam in the pool, watched movies, and got to eat seemingly any food he asked for. His mom came to visit on Sundays. Then, one day, the nurses tried to draw blood to run some tests, and Paul panicked. When he resisted, several big, male nurses came in and strapped him to the hospital table. Paul, terrified, decided he didn't like the hospital. He blamed his mother for not being there to protect him.

That day, the doctors gave Paul some pills they said would make him feel better. Paul thought that made sense. If he was at the hospital, he must be sick, and if you were sick, you got medicine, right? The medicine, though he didn't know it at the time, was Ritalin, which was meant to tamp down his hyperactivity.

If childhood depression remained largely under the radar when Claire began treatment in the early 1990s, attention deficit/hyperactivity disorder was not. Already, the condition was linked in the public consciousness with boisterous and defiant grade school boys and with the drug used to treat them: Ritalin. Ritalin had in fact been on the market since the mid-1950s to treat children who were labeled in various ways—"minimal brain dysfunction," "hyperkinetic reaction of childhood," "hyperactive child syndrome," among others—but in the late 1980s, several factors converged that bolstered the drug's popularity. An increase in diagnoses undoubtedly played a major role. In 1980, the year that the *DSM-III* renamed the condition "attention deficit disorder" and allowed for a variant that didn't include hyperactivity, an estimated quarter million to half million children were taking stimulants. In 1987, when a revised version of the manual—*DSM-III-R*—changed the disorder's name to "attention deficit/hyperactivity disorder" and simplified the diagnostic criteria, an estimated 750,000 were taking stimulants (both estimates, were, however, extrapolated based on prevalence data from local surveys).[13]

Ritalin had already assumed a big enough presence by the late 1980s to warrant a backlash. A radically antipsychiatry group affiliated with the Church of Scientology filed a spate of lawsuits against schools and doctors for allegedly pushing medication on children, and a rash of news reports raised questions about overprescribing. A neuroimaging study conducted by the National Institute of Mental Health in 1990 seemed to pave the way for more judicious prescribing when it showed decreased activity in the brain regions that regulate attention and motor control. The findings led to raised hopes that a brain scan could eventually test for the presence of ADHD, and *Time* magazine declared that "the link between brain chemistry and behavior now seems certain."[14] Needless to say, that test was not forthcoming. During the next few years, various researchers reported two- to threefold increases in the percentage of children prescribed Ritalin, so that by 1995, about 1.5 million children, or nearly 3 percent of the U.S. school-age population, was taking the drug.[15]

Ritalin and similar medications were used not only to treat attention deficit disorder, but also to curb the aggressive and hyperactive behavior found in "conduct disorder" and "oppositional defiant disorder," two more behavior diagnoses that gained traction in the 1990s. During that decade, the public's image of a child medicated for ADHD and other behavioral problems was usually male, white, and middle or upper-middle class, although data would emerge later that complicated that picture. And there was another population of kids who, it turned out, were receiving Ritalin and other behavioral medications in disproportionate numbers: foster children.

Paul entered foster care, and with it, the web of Florida's public mental health services, in 1993. It wasn't until the end of the decade that researchers began looking closely at psychotropic drug use in the foster-care system and media reports began to raise alarms over the widespread "drugging" of foster children in California, Washington, and other states. By 1993, however, numerous long-term studies had already documented significantly higher rates of emotional and behavioral problems in foster kids than in the general child population. Foster children, after all, were wards of the state precisely because they had been abused or neglected, and child development research and population studies made it clear that early trauma, abuse, or neglect put children at an increased risk of mental illness. A group of leading foster-care researchers called the system in 1997 "an open air mental hospital" unequipped to deal with such severely abused and neglected children.[16] Meanwhile, the foster-care population swelled—from a little over a quarter million children nationwide in 1982 to nearly a half million in 1994—and the number of available homes declined as potential foster parents tired of dealing with large, impenetrable state bureaucracies.[17]

The child welfare workers who placed Paul in his first foster home told him they'd taken him from his parents to put him in a safer environment. To be sure, the neighborhood was better, but Paul's new home didn't feel any safer to him because Paul's foster parents made it clear that he wasn't part of the family, and that the government paid them to care for him. Shortly after he arrived, the parents took their own children to Disney World and placed Paul in a short-term "respite" home. After they returned, the kids bragged about how much fun they'd had at Disney World. Paul, jealous and missing his parents, couldn't take that, so he ran straight out the door.

He spent most of the day on the streets, as he had done at home. He asked passersby for quarters, saying he needed them to call his mom, when really he just wanted to buy sodas. He knew one of the buses would take him to his parents, but he had no idea which one. After several hours, the police found him and dragged him back to child welfare headquarters. That would be the first of many times Paul ran away from a foster-care home he didn't like.

Over the next couple of years, he bounced through more placements, both in individual families and group homes. He struck his case manager and foster parents as a bright and charming little boy, but one intent on defying adults and asserting his dominance over other kids. The more placements he was given, the more violent and aggressive his behavior seemed to get. He beat up other children frequently, climbed up on the roof and threatened to jump and, of course, frequently ran away. His behavior quickly got him identified as a child who needed special care, and he was assigned a succession of therapists, a new one with each new placement. Despite the therapy, no one explicitly explained his medication to him, at least not in terms he could understand. Over time, though, he gleaned that it was to control his bad behavior. Sometimes, he'd be acting up, and one of his foster parents would say, "Oh, *that's* why. I forgot your medication." Or, he'd be bouncing off the walls, and they'd give him extra pills so he'd calm down and stop bothering them. Paul himself didn't notice any change in his behavior when he took Ritalin. At the group homes where he was placed, a lot of the kids were taking meds. It seemed to Paul that the more pills you were on, the more messed up you were.

Claire, ages eleven to twelve
HUDSON, OHIO / 1991–1992

About a week after she began taking a tricyclic antidepressant for her suicidal thoughts and violent mood swings, Claire Frese seemed to improve markedly. But after a few more weeks, she seemed to grow even more disturbed. It was hard to say if she had experienced something of a placebo effect at first, or whether she had quickly developed a tolerance to the medication. Adjusting the dosage over the course of several months didn't help. On a second antidepressant, Claire showed the same promising initial response but relapsed after a few months. Her meltdowns were more dramatic than ever. She'd scream at the top of her lungs in the middle of the living room, throw glasses across the kitchen, and stomp on the floor so hard her mother was afraid she'd break her ankles. Her older brother and younger sister would run for cover when she lunged at them. In a family where even roughhousing was off-limits, Claire's behavior was distinctly unacceptable—and she knew it. "The medication isn't working," her parents told her. "We need to find another one that works better."

After six months of therapy and tricyclic antidepressants from the family pediatrician, Claire's parents managed to wrangle a referral to see a child psychiatrist. Then they spent another three months waiting for an appointment. That was hardly unusual. At the time Ohio had about one child psychiatrist for every twenty-three thousand children, right around the national median, but still far less than many medical advocacy groups considered sufficient.[18] In 1990 the American Academy of Child and Adolescent Psychiatry called for a big education push to train more specialists, but the additional years of training required, combined with low reimbursement rates compared to other medical specialties and the difficulty of treating children with a then-limited arsenal of medications, made it hard to recruit enough clinicians. The shortage persists today.

Having spent nine months watching Claire flounder on her current medication regimen, Fred and Penny went to the psychiatrist appointment knowing exactly what they wanted. Like much of the rest of the country, they had read and heard a lot about the new antidepressant Prozac. The drug, which had come on the U.S. market in 1988, was in a new class of antidepressants called selective serotonin reuptake inhibitors because they specifically target the brain neurotransmitter serotonin. The older antidepressants, including the tricyclics like those Claire had tried, affect multiple neurotransmitter systems; because Prozac is "selective," it was supposed to be more effective and also produce fewer and apparently less severe side effects. Fred had seen Prozac work wonders for some of his adult patients, and his daughter from his first marriage seemed to be doing better on it, too, after sinking into a severe depression during her freshman year in college. Fred and Penny resolved to ask the new psychiatrist if he'd write Claire a prescription.

Despite the buzz about Prozac as the new wonder drug for depression and a range of other conditions from anxiety disorders to severe PMS and eating disorders, information in 1991 about its safety and effectiveness for children was next to nonexistent. Doctors who prescribed it to children had little to go on but some scattered published case reports, anecdotal information from colleagues, or gut instinct that what worked for adults might work for kids, too. Few clinicians were ready to take the risk. Indeed, when statistics about antidepressant prescribing trends in children finally became available a decade later, they would show that just one in a thousand children with a managed care plan like Claire's received an SSRI in 1991, though that figure would increase sixfold just three years later and would continue to rise dramatically for the next decade.[19] Overall, between 1988, the year Prozac came on the U.S. market, and 1994, there was a nineteenfold increase in the number of children prescribed an SSRI.[20] A survey of some twelve hundred child psychiatrists in 1996 and 1997 found SSRIs to be the drug treatment of choice for children under twelve with depression.[21] But when Claire's parents made their request, the psychiatrist emphasized that the drug had no track record in children, and he made them sign a waiver acknowledging they understood what he told them. Then he wrote the script.

Elizabeth, age twelve
WASHINGTON, DC, SUBURBS / 1993

Life in twelve-year-old Elizabeth's house in an affluent Maryland suburb of DC had never been peaceful, but by the fall of 1993, her parents' marriage was falling apart, and she was taking it hard before she even knew quite what was happening.

The family had started therapy the summer after she finished sixth grade, and while Liz did not understand why, she did know one thing: she didn't want to be there. In the early sessions, she spoke only when asked a direct question, perhaps because she was confused by the situation, or perhaps because by the time she was twelve, Liz had already somehow picked up on the stigma often associated with seeing a therapist—it meant there was something wrong with you. By this time, her mother had already noticed that she seemed less self-confident and needier, wanting her mother to be with her, especially when she was doing homework. When her mom suggested that Liz might want to talk to the counselor at her elementary school, pointing out that her best friend, whose parents were splitting up, had been going weekly, Liz refused.

Unlike Claire, who was not particularly forthcoming in therapy but who didn't hide things from her parents, Liz, mirroring her father, avoided discussing her troubles both in therapy and at home. In therapy, discussions sometimes centered on her lack of participation in the sessions, and she felt like her every move was being analyzed. If she kicked at her father's feet or made faces at her nineteen-year-old sister, it signified a desire to connect. When she folded her arms across her chest or looked at the floor, she was attempting to remove herself from the proceedings.

During the following holiday season, when her sister came home for Christmas, her parents sat them down and explained that her father had been depressed and would be moving out of the house. They didn't say anything about the real reasons for the separation: her mother, who had already endured years of her husband's alcoholism, recovery, and relapses, had discovered that he was having an affair and had given him an ultimatum, demanding he choose between her and his mistress. During their annual post-Christmas family vacation in Florida that year, Liz noticed that her older sister was furious with their father but not their mother, and concluded that whatever had happened must be their dad's fault. Like a lot of kids whose parents split up, she also felt that the responsibility somehow lay with her. One day she told her mother, sobbing, that she would do her homework and stop yelling and be better if her parents would just get back together.

The family kept up therapy after Liz's dad moved out, but they still didn't talk about the reasons for her parents' separation. Instead, when they went to therapy, Liz's parents and sister, who came to sessions during her college breaks, seemed to spend the entire time discussing Liz—how she refused to do any chores, how she had screaming fights with her parents, how she'd taken to cursing, how she finished her homework late at night or not at all. Years later, when Liz studied psychology in college, it would occur to her that she was, in the parlance of family systems theory, the "designated patient," the one whose problems stood in for the dysfunction of the whole family.

While her family analyzed her problem behavior at their sessions, she'd sit mutely. At home, she had for years driven her family crazy with her nonstop chatter, but as things grew more tense between her parents, she talked less and less, except during the blowups with her parents. When her sister called home from college, all she'd get from Liz were one-word answers. "How are you doing, Liz?" "Fine." "How are things at home?" "Weird." No matter how much her sister pushed, "weird" was as far as Liz's descriptions ever got for a couple of years. Once, her sister told Liz she was being just like their dad—unwilling to talk about her emotions. That stuck with her.

For seventh grade, Liz had switched from public elementary school to the elite DC private school her sister had attended. In elementary school, Liz had alternated between spacing out in class and worrying about being called on and embarrassed in front of her peers. "Please don't call on me, please don't call on me, please don't call on me," she'd repeat over and over in her head, even when she knew the answer. She procrastinated on her homework and often ended up doing it late at night in a panic with a friend who was as disorganized as she was and whose parents were similarly laid-back about rules and bedtimes. Still, she always managed to make good grades, and was something of a teacher's pet. At Liz's new school, the teachers didn't go through a checklist of names when students submitted their assignments, which saved Liz the embarrassment of being scolded in front of her classmates. She stopped doing any homework she couldn't finish during class. At home, it was just too difficult to focus. When called on in class, she didn't know even the easy answers, and when the teachers chewed her out in front of her classmates, she cried. She spent lunchtimes reading, alone.

Liz had had headaches for as long as she could remember, but by seventh grade they were getting worse, and she was also complaining more frequently of stomachaches and other vague ailments. Her mother, who had taken Liz to the pediatrician about her headaches many times over the years and had a large collection of child and family psychology books around the house, eventually concluded that the aches and pains must be psychosomatic. "Elizabeth, you're just feeling sick because you're worried about school," she'd say, when Liz tried to get out of attending. Her mom's rule was that she wasn't allowed to miss school unless she had a fever, but in practice she missed a good deal of school because she was just too worked up to attend and her mother did not insist.

Because Liz wasn't turning in any homework and seemed depressed after her father moved out, her mother thought she should see her own therapist in addition to the ongoing family therapy. Liz, who was shy with strangers, insisted her mother accompany her to sessions. But that provided only so much protection. The therapists tended to ask big, open-ended questions Liz had no idea how to answer: "So, why do you think you're here?" Liz would refuse to answer any questions about her parents, her feelings, or her thoughts on why she was in therapy. Inevitably, she'd go through a session or two, complain to her mom that she hated the counselor and therapy in general, and get a temporary reprieve from appointments. Eventually, her mother would find her a new therapist, and the cycle would begin again.

Her mother, wracked with anxiety over her marriage falling apart and—though Liz didn't know it at the time—over her husband's infidelity and alcoholism, was at a loss. She kept Liz's dad in the loop, but he was a busy lawyer at a high-powered firm and had never been much involved in parenting decisions. At one point in seventh grade, Liz's mother had a doctor prescribe some pills that she told her daughter were for headaches. Her mom made sure she took a pill a day for a week or two, but when Liz developed a rash on her leg, her mother got nervous, called the doctor, and took her off the medication. Liz wouldn't find out until more than a decade later that she'd been taking antidepressants.

Claire, Paul, and Liz all initially got into treatment—and on meds—because, to varying degrees, they externalized their problems and thus became identified as "problem kids." Children who disturb the peace at home or school are more likely to get noticed in any era, but whereas in past decades parents, teachers, and doctors tended to consider these kids as merely unruly or delinquent, in the 1990s, they were more likely to identify the problem as a symptom of a diagnosable mental disorder that, crucially, could be treated with medication. The majority of these children, especially boys like Paul, were diagnosed with ADHD and treated with stimulants like Ritalin. Others, especially girls like Liz and Claire, who were less hyperactive and considered more "emotional," were more likely to get an antidepressant, although as the 1990s came to a close, the ratio of girls to boys taking stimulants would even out somewhat.

Perhaps just as important as the diagnosis they received or the drugs they were prescribed, though, are the circumstances under which they received their medication. Paul, Liz, and Claire all entered medication treatment at a time when they were too young or too recalcitrant to ask for help themselves. Their problems were something grown-ups decided needed fixing. In Claire's case, her parents explained medication to her in more sophisticated terms than many doctors would have used—as a potentially effective treatment but not a cure, as something that would help ease the symptoms of her depression but that she would probably need to take in one form or another for the rest of her life. In the absence of a clear explanation for treatment or a good grasp of their problems to begin with, though, children are left to piece things together as best they can. Paul, given Ritalin at age five with scarcely any explanation, struggled to make sense of the fact that even though he was supposedly a "bad" kid and the medications were supposed to help him control his anger, the pills didn't seem to change his behavior or his emotions. Liz, meanwhile, got conflicting messages about the nature of her problems and wasn't even told she was taking an antidepressant. This wasn't the end of the story for Liz, or for Paul or Claire. It was only the beginning of a long, complicated, and often dramatic process of forging a relationship with medication and understanding its powerful impact.

CHAPTER 2

Playing a Role
The Medicated Kid

Claire, ages thirteen to fourteen
HUDSON, OHIO / 1994–1995

My name is Claire Frese. I'm thirteen years old. I have a good
number of friends, I guess, although sometimes I think nobody
likes me. They're all the most interesting people a person could
ever meet. They're all really important to me. We like to spend
time together. We go to the library after school and then walk to
McDonald's for a sundae. Sometimes we have sleepovers or hang
out together. Otherwise we spend hours on the phone. It drives
my mom crazy, but she knows it's all part of growing up. Another
part of growing up, for me, is learning to live with my disability.
I have depression.

This is the opening voice-over of *Claire's Story*, Claire's educational film
about childhood depression, which was eventually incorporated into the
curricula of health classes around Ohio. Accompanying the voice-over
are shots of Claire and her friends at McDonald's, giggling and gossiping about a boy who has a crush on Claire, followed by a long take of

them skipping down the picturesque main street of Claire's hometown and peeking into the window of a toy store. The music is resolutely upbeat. Years later, Claire and her mother couldn't agree exactly on how they decided to make the film, but the story her mother liked to tell was that Claire, though her own problems were under control, worried about some friends who seemed to be exhibiting symptoms of depression but weren't getting help. Fred and Penny had recently made a video of their own discussing how the family learned to cope with Fred's schizophrenia; after they showed it at mental health conferences, orders had poured in. It occurred to Penny that there was probably at least as much hunger for a child's personal take on depression. School health classes at the time rarely discussed mental illness, and if they did, it was generally limited to a brief mention of suicide prevention. Penny thought children should be taught to recognize depression before they got desperate enough to contemplate killing themselves.

Claire loved making the film. She had acted in school plays and relished the chance to write her own lines and weigh in on the overall script. Starring in her own movie also gave her a certain cachet with her peers—and she got to miss two weeks of school to boot. Some of the scenes were filmed at her school, which added to her mystique. *Claire's Story* would be the first of her many appearances as a poster child for youth depression and pharmaceutical treatment—a role she played gamely and enthusiastically for the next several years.

Though few of Claire's peers adopted the role of "medicated child" so knowingly, her experience was in many ways typical. Deeply disturbed children used to be permanently institutionalized or at least hospitalized for long stays, while those with less debilitating troubles often received no care at all. As part of the first generation of young people to remain fully integrated into their families, schools, and communities while receiving medical treatment for psychiatric disorders, Claire and her peers had few models to fashion themselves after. To a large extent, like Claire, they were writing their own roles, though with substantial input and influence from their parents, doctors, siblings, peers, and teachers. Being diagnosed with a mental illness and being treated with medication, to a far greater extent than these kids could foresee when they took their first pill, would have a deep and lasting impact on how they viewed themselves. To be sure, before going on medication, some children and teenagers worried about side effects, and child psychiatrists described to me some particularly self-aware young patients brooding over how the drugs might change their identities. For the most part, though, they took the drugs unthinkingly, perhaps a little nervously, reluctantly, or angrily, but, kids being classic short-term thinkers, without considering quite what they were getting themselves into. Certainly they didn't contemplate that ten or twenty years later they might still be sorting out the effects the drugs had had—and would have—on them.

The medications almost immediately became a fixture in these children's lives and demanded a shift in self-assessment and self-definition. The fact is that for the purposes of ongoing treatment, a pill isn't just a pill. Taking drugs as prescribed, as a number of medical anthropologists argue, requires an ongoing process of interpretation and justification: What purpose is the medication supposed to serve, and how well is it serving that purpose? The imprecision of psychiatric diagnosis and the difficulty of gauging medications' effectiveness make answering those questions difficult in any context. For children and teenagers, who are often given incomplete or confusing explanations of their conditions and how their drugs work, the task becomes even more complex. Their assessment of the drug's purpose and how well it serves that purpose can be as mercurial as their rapidly changing moods. Sometimes, the transformation is evident to them shortly after beginning medication; sometimes it takes much longer to sort out why they needed medication, to what extent it has worked, and what that means for their developing identities.

By emphasizing the sheer normality of Claire's life, *Claire's Story* helped clarify the first point, the reasons for taking medication. After the opening shots of her cavorting with her friends, the camera switched to a rollicking scene of the family building a snowman in front of their big, white house. The voice-over, in Claire's midwestern accent and teenage intonation, tells viewers, "I like my family. I like my house and town. And even my school is pretty cool, for a school, anyway. So what is there to be depressed about? That's just it," she continues. "I'm not depressed about *something*. I'm just depressed, and it could be anything that any other day wouldn't bother me at all."

Released in 1995, *Claire's Story* reflects the ethos of the time, a time when scientists seemed on the verge of discovering the secrets of the brain and, potentially, the roots of mental illness. Referencing the flurry of excitement about neuroscience findings that was beginning to define the decade, a stentorian voice-over intones, "The 1990s have been called the Decade of the Brain." The film emphasizes the hopefulness inherent in the zeitgeist. "I have depression, but that doesn't mean I'm miserable," Claire told viewers. "Depression is not a disease—it's a condition. It can last for a few weeks, months, or even your whole life. Because it's a medical problem, it needs medical treatment." Often, the adult narrator adds, that means psychotropic medication. At this point, Claire pops in cheerily to translate, "Those are medications that help the brain to work properly."

Claire's mother, Penny, had made a point in the film to describe depression as "a condition" because she thought referring to depression as a disease, an increasingly common tactic in some advocacy circles, marked sufferers as sick and permanently damaged. She didn't want Claire or other children to think of depression as a life sentence of misery because doing so might leave them feeling helpless or hopeless. Rather, the film emphasizes the active role children can take in interpreting their treatment, describing how Claire was on the lookout for side effects and recurring symptoms. The film also features interviews with Claire's friends in which they talk about accepting her for who she is, depressed or not.

Claire was the first of the three younger Frese children to be diagnosed and medicated for depression; in short order, both her older brother Joe and her younger sister Bridget would also be prescribed SSRIs. Claire's poise and good humor made her an appealing poster child, though her brother Joe's dramatic recovery underscored the ways in which Claire's real story did not, in fact, have a neat ending.

Joe, two years older than Claire, was in tenth grade when he helped his mother and sister shoot *Claire's Story*. He'd been bogged down in apathy and gloom since fifth grade, when it had dawned on him that there was a social pecking order, and that his social circle was quite definitely stuck near the bottom. Hanging out with his nerdy friends seemed pointless and moving up the social ladder impossible, so he started spending most of his time alone. He transferred to a Jesuit boys' school near the Freses' home in suburban Cleveland, but after an unhappy, socially isolated ninth grade year, his parents switched him back to the public high school. Despite having helped Claire and Penny write and prepare *Claire's Story*—the credits list him as assistant director—Joe didn't think his unhappiness, or even his occasional thoughts of suicide, qualified him as depressed. To him, these only marked him as pathetic.

With a schizophrenic husband and two daughters diagnosed with depression, his mother had enough experience to suspect otherwise. Joe had been a mild-mannered, easygoing kid, quite different from Claire. For him to turn into a hermit who grunted rather than spoke seemed too extreme for ordinary adolescent angst. One day during his sophomore year, Penny went up to Joe's bedroom, where he spent nearly all his free time, and found him curled up in a fetal position on his bed. She read him a checklist of depression symptoms and asked, "Joe, do any of these apply to you?" For once, she got more than a grunt. "All of them," Joe said. "Including thinking about suicide."

Penny had made *Claire's Story* in part to make sure kids got help before suicide entered the picture. She felt terrible. But this time, she and Fred resolved to do things differently—no more treading water in therapy waiting for their HMO to authorize a referral to a child psychiatrist. Penny called the insurance people and said, "I can send him to a therapist, but two of his sisters are already on medication—you'll be wasting your money." The company gave in. Joe didn't need any convincing to see the psychiatrist. As soon as he realized other people thought his symptoms were severe enough to warrant treatment, his self-reproach and guilt lifted.

Given his parents' pro-medication bent and Claire's experience, Joe wasn't surprised when the psychiatrist, the same one whom Claire saw,

diagnosed him with depression and prescribed Zoloft—a new drug that
had come on the market a couple of years earlier and had been approved
for treating depression in adults. Like Prozac, Zoloft was a selective
serotonin reuptake inhibitor, or SSRI, which was supposed to work on
more specific brain pathways than the older drugs and also to have
fewer and milder side effects. What did surprise Joe was just how rapidly
and dramatically he improved. Although Prozac had evened out Claire's
most dramatic rages and weeping fits, she continued to have considerable trouble sleeping and some difficulty modulating her emotions.
Zoloft seemed to make Joe into someone else altogether, a remarkably
well-adjusted teenager. All of a sudden, and seemingly without trying,
he had a group of friends, and was laughing with them a lot. At the first
school drama club meeting he attended, he was elected club president,
much to Claire's frustration since she had been faithfully attending
meeting after meeting. Soon, Joe was getting parts in plays and elected
a class officer. He didn't spend a lot of time thinking about how he used
to be depressed, but, having grown up in a family where mental illnesses
were viewed as biological disorders, he understood his current happiness as a logical consequence of medical treatment.

Joe's reaction to Zoloft sounds like a classic account of the wonders
of the SSRIs, the sort of miracle turnaround story that made Prozac a
blockbuster for its maker, Eli Lilly, and that was also rapidly making
Zoloft a major moneymaker for Lilly's rival, Pfizer. In 1993, the same
year Joe went on medication, the psychiatrist Peter Kramer published
the best-selling *Listening to Prozac*, which examined the phenomenon
of patients who seemed to become "better than well"—more energetic,
more assertive, more ambitious than they'd ever been. Kramer wondered if these startling by-products of medication would encourage
"cosmetic psychopharmacology," a term he coined to describe people
taking medications to rid themselves of personality traits our driven,
competitive culture discourages and to enhance those that society
rewards.[1]

Mostly, Kramer described adults who, like those profiled in news
stories and television specials about the new antidepressants, found sal-
vation after suffering from mental illness for years, or had lived happy,

productive lives before being struck by pathological symptoms. He brings up young people only in his discussion of Prozac's fascinating ability to reduce what he terms "rejection-sensitivity," a term for intense insecurity and desire for social approval. Briefly, he notes his reluctance to prescribe medication for his "rejection-sensitive" college students, given his conviction that short-term psychotherapy was perfectly suited to such cases. Kramer said he might be willing to consider a course of medication for a student undergoing a protracted depression, or one who was so sensitive and vulnerable that he or she could not function, interact normally with peers, or maintain a healthy sense of self-worth. For the most part, though, in *Listening to Prozac*, Kramer left the notion of medicating young people firmly in the realm of the hypothetical.

Joe, arguably, had experienced the problems Kramer described, though they had come on so gradually that he thought he was just having a rough adolescence. With Zoloft, however, he felt transformed. His quick and dramatic response, validated by his sudden popularity, provided a solid logical framework on which to base his understanding of both his illness and his treatment: the medication corrected a biological problem in his brain. End of story. While Kramer and others were debating the ethics of remaking one's personality with medication, Joe was just happy to be well.

His lack of self-questioning wasn't, I think, surprising. As long as there are no troublesome side effects, most young people like Joe who experience a clear and unambiguous improvement in their mood and behavior are happy to accept their medication with little self-questioning. Speaking from experience, I can say that medication at its best enables you to feel that you are playing the role you were always meant to play.

Despite the dominant narrative in the late '80s and early '90s that medication, especially SSRIs, could be transformative, medication did not, of course, work so neatly or perfectly for everyone. Compared to Joe and their little sister Bridget, who a year later at age twelve also had a strong and unambiguously positive response to an SSRI, Claire's was a more qualified success story. Two years before Joe's about-face, Claire hadn't responded well to the two tricyclic antidepressants her pediatrician prescribed. Later, Prozac failed to erase either her insomnia or her daytime exhaustion. Then, after a year or two, her emotional meltdowns returned in full force, so her doctor switched her to Zoloft. For years after that, Claire would alternate between Prozac and Zoloft, returning to one when the other seemed to lose its potency. As soon as she began taking medication, her parents had explained—with a degree of nuance and honesty many adults probably wouldn't use with an eleven-year-old—that it was important to be patient and continue looking for a drug that would help her. Thus Claire learned from an early age that drugs were not inevitable panaceas. Medication had helped her father live a remarkably productive life despite his schizophrenia, but he still had relapses, still had to contend with side effects. Such was the nature of psychiatric treatment, unless, of course, you were lucky enough to be someone like Joe.

In fact, that SSRIs worked so dramatically for her brother and sister only seemed to reinforce the relative severity of Claire's problems. "I'm the *real* kid with depression," she would sometimes think to herself. Her depression couldn't be eliminated in one fell swoop with a pill; it was complicated and intractable and required constant tending.

Claire's burgeoning role as a teen mental health advocate also helped reinforce the legitimacy of her illness and the importance of vigilant treatment. *Claire's Story* was picked up by several area schools, and was later included in the statewide health curriculum. Through high school and into college, Claire was quoted by regional and national media in stories on youth depression and medication. Discussing her experience again and again, she kept circling back to how she'd been before, reminding herself in the process that she really was better after all, thanks primarily to medication.

Claire's experience speaks to the need for young people on medication to contend with two separate yet interrelated concepts: having a brain-based disorder and requiring medication to treat that disorder. In a culture that has now widely embraced the "chemical imbalance" theory of mental illness, the two might seem inextricably linked. But at the time Claire started taking SSRIs parents and doctors often avoided linking the medicine too closely to a specific diagnosis, for fear of "labeling." In part, this had to do with the ethos of the time, for the 1980s and 1990s were the great era of political correctness, when schoolchildren were taught to say "mentally challenged" rather than "retarded," when everybody was, in the great euphemism of the time, "special." The worst thing you could do to a child, it seemed, was crush her self-esteem—or give her a label that would prevent her from achieving her dreams, however improbable those dreams might be. Critics of the increase in children being diagnosed and treated for psychiatric problems often invoked this line of reasoning. A 1993 article from the *Journal of Child and Adolescent Psychiatric Nursing*, concerned with the particular danger of labeling minority children, summed up the sentiment well: "The DSM psychiatric diagnostic system created its own self-fulfilling prophesies, stigmatizing children with lifelong images of being damaged, defective, and intractible."[2]

DSM diagnoses could be downplayed, however. The model of mental illness as a chemical imbalance, which was heavily promoted in the television ads for psychiatric meds that began airing in the late 1990s, particularly suited the no-blame, empowerment ethos of the self-esteem movement. Rather than emphasizing "depression" or "attention deficit disorder" as separate and potentially powerful forces that defined the child, the problem was reduced to something more generic and benign-sounding. By separating the child from the problem, the chemical imbalance model allowed children, potentially, to transcend their illness, just as the disability rights movement encouraged people to proclaim, "I am not my disability."

The fact was, however, that children were being labeled more than ever before, given ever more specific diagnoses, and often more than one diagnosis at a time for multiple disorders, a phenomenon doctors call comorbidity. The labels weren't always conveyed to the kids, however, either because doctors or parents feared saddling them with an illness that might make them feel different or less capable than their peers, or because the diagnoses themselves were inherently uncertain. Even as new versions of the *DSM* identified more and more conditions as pathological, there was heated debate within the psychiatric profession over how to classify disorders, a debate that continues to this day as the profession argues fiercely about the latest revision of the manual, the *DSM-V*, due out in 2013.

Childhood disorders have been among the most controversial psychiatric diagnoses, in part because of the inherent difficulties of distinguishing pathology from normal development. Insurance companies often require a diagnosis for reimbursement, but doctors did, and still do, enter diagnosis codes with a considerable degree of skepticism. Since there is no definitive biological test to verify the existence of a disorder or to distinguish one condition from another, diagnoses tend to shift over time. Psychiatrists I interviewed who have been practicing at least since the late 1980s described being reluctant to tell young children that they had a given condition, because of the uncertainty of diagnosis and the potential for symptoms to change. But a number of them emphasized the importance of explaining to a child the reasons for medication, in part because children often worry that medication will harm them, and interpret the pills as a sign that they are defective or damaged.

Despite pervasive fears about their potential to stigmatize, labels aren't intrinsically bad. Some kids do long for an explanation for their being different, says the eminent ADHD researcher and child psychiatrist Glen Elliott. As he put it, "A label can sometimes be a very potent answer to that very frustrating dilemma." Sometimes, naming and identifying the problem make it easier to perform the constant interpretive process that Jeffrey Longhofer and Jerry Floersch, social workers and academics who study adolescents' experience of psychotropic meds, call "the daily work of being medicated." This process of comparison between the before-medication and after-medication selves, they argue, is what kids use to justify the need for psychopharmaceutical treatment.[3] And ongoing treatment, with all its hassles and downsides, certainly needs justification. It needn't be a *DSM* label, but kids need some means of understanding the nature of the problems that medication is supposed to fix. In a study of St. Louis teenagers who received public mental health services, for example, the researcher Tally Moses found that four out of five kids were unsure or confused about how to characterize their problems, but that those who self-identified as having a psychiatric disorder were nearly six times as likely to report a strong commitment to continuing their medications than those who didn't self-identify that way.[4] Other studies have also found that a diagnosis justifies the need for medication.[5] But a label alone isn't necessarily enough for kids struggling to understand the nature of their problems and the reasons for drug treatment. Elizabeth, for one, spent several years confused about just what, exactly, was wrong with her, and a diagnosis and two prescriptions did little to clear that up.

Elizabeth, ages thirteen to fourteen
WASHINGTON, DC, SUBURBS / 1994–1995

A few months after Elizabeth's mother gave her antidepressants disguised as headache medication, her mom arranged, on the advice of her own therapist, with whom Liz had met several times, for Liz to have a formal evaluation for learning, attention, and emotional troubles. Perhaps because Liz was so averse to discussing her emotions, both Liz's mom and the psychologist framed the testing as a way to find out why Liz might be faring poorly in school. Almost as soon as the test began, however, Liz could see that it was something more than a measure of academic aptitude. She felt tricked. She answered the questions that had to do with schoolwork, but boycotted the inkblot interpretations and anything that seemed like an attempt to get at her feelings. The report suggested that she was anxious and ill-equipped to handle stress. Instead, it said, she tended to lash out, act impulsively, or shut down altogether: she "presents as an adolescent of extraordinary intellectual ability who is depressed and has a mild difficulty in written expression and a mild attention deficit disorder," the report read. She "is a young lady who is in significant emotional distress, although she works hard to cover up her pain. Therapeutic work with her needs to be supportive as well as focused on helping her develop more effective coping skills." It also suggested that she see a psychiatrist for a consultation about medication for her mood disorder.

Later that summer, Liz went to sleepaway camp in New England. For the first time, she found herself around kids who didn't make a secret of how unhappy they were, who even flaunted it. A girl in her bunk talked so much about suicide that the camp confiscated the girl's aspirin and summoned her mother for an emergency visit. Liz and a friend spent a five-day hiking trip lusting after an older boy from the boys' camp next door who talked, in what struck them as an alluringly melancholic tone, about wanting to kill himself. Happy to be separated from feuding parents, probing therapists, and concerned school guidance counselors, Liz started to think about herself not just as a slacker and a disaffected teen—in seventh grade she took to listening to grunge music, relishing the profane lyrics—but as a depressed, "fucked-up" kid, an identity founded, in part, on her dysfunctional family situation. She wrote increasingly dark journal entries, and showed some passages to a few friends. Some of them seemed overawed, others a little freaked out. Upon reading Liz's emoting about her parents splitting up, one friend said, "Oh, my God. That's so *sad.*" Another friend signed a souvenir pillowcase with the words, "Enough of this death, death, death, die, die, die, stuff!"

When Liz returned to Maryland at the end of the summer, she ripped out and burned all the journal passages describing her unhappiness. She hid the pillowcase with her friend's exhortation to stop the gloom and doom. She couldn't stand the idea of her mother knowing how unhappy she was, and she didn't think her school friends cared enough about her to listen to her disturbed thoughts without laughing at her or gossiping about her. At camp, depression had seemed almost cool. Back home, it struck her, as it had Joe Frese, as simply pathetic. Liz still wrote privately in her diary about how unhappy she sometimes was, but wondered how to interpret it. Upon taking a "Could you be depressed?" quiz in the teen magazine *YM*, she noted that she sometimes felt deeply melancholic, but other times felt just a vague malaise. "I don't want to live, but I don't want to die," she wrote in her diary just before beginning eighth grade, adding, "I would *not* commit suicide." Even when she felt things were so bad that she was tempted to give up trying to hold it together, she always heard a little voice in her head saying, *Maybe it's all going to get better and be okay in a way you can't see right now.*

At the end of eighth grade, Liz narrowly escaped being "asked" to withdraw from her elite private school. She also continued to suffer from bad headaches most days, and at the beginning of ninth grade, her mother announced they were going to a psychiatrist to see if anything could be done to reduce her stress and eliminate her headaches. The doctor asked a lot of questions about her ability to focus, and Liz, who had read an article about ADHD in one of the newsweeklies her mother subscribed to, guessed pretty quickly what the doctor was targeting. At one point, she noticed she was tapping her foot and wondered if the psychiatrist would take it as a sign of hyperactivity.

In the end, the doctor prescribed Ritalin and Prozac. She wasn't particularly clear on his reasons for giving her the latter except that for some reason he thought people tended to get depressed after going on Ritalin. Perhaps that was his logic, but he may have also thought Liz was already depressed, either because of her poor academic performance or her parents' marital troubles, and could benefit from an antidepressant. *Driven to Distraction*, a best-selling book on ADHD that had come out the previous year, emphasized that the conditions overlapped and that academic failure could send some people into a low-level depression.[6] It's also possible, though, that either the doctor or Liz's mother thought that telling her they were treating her only for ADHD, not depression, would make Liz feel better about taking an antidepressant.

On one level, Liz was glad to have the ADHD diagnosis. It was better than being dismissed as bratty and difficult, or lazy and underachieving—certainly less humiliating than nearly failing school because she couldn't focus enough to complete her homework. On the other hand, she'd read quite a bit about ADHD, and wondered if she'd tricked the doctor into prescribing a drug she didn't really need. Nevertheless, she was happy to take Ritalin if it would help her in school. Had she known irritability was a sign of depression in kids, she likely would have hoped very much for the Prozac to work; she hated losing control and getting into fights with her parents all the time. As it was, she figured that taking meds was easier than stonewalling her way through one therapy appointment after another and discussing her feelings with her mother, which she found excruciating. She figured that if she just took the pills and didn't act depressed around her parents, the fuss would end.

In fact, the fuss did end—and that was the problem. Liz's parents had been absent—"either literally or metaphorically," as she put it to me years later—for much of her childhood, and when she began to exhibit problem behavior, they didn't do much to help her figure out what exactly was wrong. They certainly worried about her and took steps to try to help, but they were so preoccupied with their own troubles that they generally didn't follow up on those measures and kept Liz in the dark about the results of her evaluation. When she did go on medication, then, she wasn't sure of the reasons for doing so, and the psychiatrist did little to clear up her confusion. All this set her up for what would be a tenuous relationship with medication.

Looking back many years later, it seemed odd to Liz that she had been given two drugs at once—one as a "just in case" measure to protect against depression. Usually, clinicians consider it wise to start a child, or an adult for that matter, on one drug at a time, so that any side effects or bad reactions will be clearly attributable to a single medication. But the prevalence of comorbidity and a growing tendency to augment one drug with another to achieve certain desired outcomes—a stimulant for focusing during the day and a sleeping medication to counteract the activating effects of the stimulant at night, for example—often resulted in more kids being on multiple medications at once during the 1990s. Of those kids who took psychotropic meds in 1987, 4.7 percent took more than one drug. That number had grown to 11.6 percent by 1996, although it's important to note that this figure still represents a tiny fraction of the overall youth population.[7] Between 1996 and 2007, the proportion of children's outpatient medication visits in which more than one psychotropic was prescribed rose from one in seven to one in five. Most of the multiple-drug prescribing, however, was done by psychiatrists rather than general practitioners and involved older children and teenagers with multiple diagnoses, presumably indicating they had more severe or complex cases.[8] Prescribing antidepressants and stimulants together, as Liz's doctor did, also increased in the mid-1990s: one study of doctor's office visits found that the drugs went from being prescribed together 4 percent of the time in 1994 to 29 percent in 1997, a sevenfold increase.[9] Since multiple drugs may be prescribed to treat a single disorder, to counteract side effects of another medication, or to treat multiple disorders, one can see how kids might have trouble figuring out just what the connection was between their problems and their meds.

Although more kids were getting drugs, and more drugs at once, few were simultaneously receiving therapy. A national study of U.S. doctors' office visits found that just 11 percent of visits by children aged nineteen and under involved therapy in addition to psychotropic treatment.[10] This resembled trends in the adult population, though overall, fewer children than adults received therapy.[11] The decrease was largely driven by insurance companies' policies of reimbursing doctors more per minute for medication consultations than for therapy and of limiting coverage of psychotherapy visits.[12] Even the lucky people who could afford dual treatment, like Liz's family, often weren't motivated to pursue it, since the meds had a way of making therapy seem redundant, or at least not so necessary. Liz found that after she went on Ritalin and Prozac, her mother didn't press the issue of therapy. Simply knowing Liz was on a medication regimen gave her mother some comfort; that her grades were improving and she was making friends was also promising. In fact, Liz, who wanted more than anything for her mother not to bug her about her depression, was making a point of not acting sullen, glum, or listless in front of her, even though she remained significantly more depressed than she let on. Her mother bought the act.

Some of Liz's medicated peers, of course, welcomed therapy. One young man named Adam received first counseling, and then both medication and therapy around the time that his older brother was diagnosed and treated for schizophrenia. His parents were preoccupied with his brother, who was vandalizing homes and committing other petty crimes, and with his older sister's leaving for college. So when they suggested that Adam see a therapist, he welcomed the chance to discuss his feelings. He felt at best lukewarm, though, about taking the antidepressant Effexor, which had come on the market a few years earlier. His role as a medicated kid was far from clear to him, in part because he never received any diagnosis or formal reason for the medication—a stark contrast to his brother's situation, which Adam could see was so grave that it clearly required chemical intervention. Adam attributed his unhappiness solely to a painful breakup back in seventh grade, and he didn't see how a pill could change his feelings. A therapist, at least, could provide a sympathetic ear.

For many kids, though, pills were more appealing precisely because they did not involve submitting the psyche to prying adult eyes. Patrick Jamieson, who now heads the Annenberg Foundation's Adolescent Mental Health Initiative, recounts having such an attitude in a combination memoir and self-help book for teens with bipolar disorder. Taking lithium and providing regular blood and urine samples to ensure that the drug didn't reach toxic levels felt invasive, but even worse, for him, was the talk therapy. "These are years in which our bedrooms are off-limits even to family members, in which phone conversations with friends take on a conspiratorial tone," he writes, quite rightly, of adolescence. To have an adult enter this "walled-off world," posing embarrassingly intimate questions about romantic feelings, friendships, sexual urges, or parent-child relationships—to be asked, in essence to be "self-reflective on command"—felt to him like a worse violation than providing blood and urine samples.[13]

As a teenager, I also viewed therapy as an egregious violation of my privacy, more invasive than even the painful and traumatic medical treatment I'd endured a couple of years earlier for scoliosis, a curvature of the spine that often worsens during adolescent growth spurts. That had been memorably unpleasant. At the beginning of seventh grade, just as I was starting middle school, I started wearing a back brace—the standard first-line treatment, meant to keep the curve from progressing and causing problems later in life. Back braces are hot, awkward, and uncomfortable, covering, at a minimum, your hips and ribcage, limiting your movement, and requiring you to wear large, bulky clothes to hide the sharp outlines of the plastic.

Wearing a brace twenty hours a day is unpleasant enough even in the best of circumstances, but it gave me such severe lesions and blisters that I could tolerate it only a few hours at a time. My curve continued to worsen, and at the end of seventh grade I was told to prepare for spinal fusion, a major operation that would have consigned me to six months of bed rest. In the end, I narrowly avoided the surgery, but the whole experience left me anxious and desperately self-conscious about my body—contributing, I suspect, to my developing an eating disorder at the beginning of high school, not to mention to my subsequent depression.

I hated the brace, and certainly didn't relish the hospital gowns, the X-rays and MRIs, or the physical therapy that accompanied the treatment. Yet, when it came to resenting adult intrusion into my life, psychotherapy for my eating disorder was far worse. Looking back, I certainly don't fault my parents for trying to get me professional help, but at the time, being made to discuss my innermost secrets, worries, and hang-ups with an adult felt like punishment, not treatment. When one therapist and then another concluded that my main problems were underlying anxiety and persistent, low-level depression, I grew hopeful, thinking this might open up the door for antidepressants that I had read worked wonders for mood disorders. But over the course of the next two years, neither of my therapists nor my parents broached the subject. I wondered why, but feared that requesting the drug myself would only invite more scrutiny.

Adults sometimes worry about giving children medication because they fear it will pose a barrier to self-reflection and better self-understanding, especially if used in lieu of therapy. In my case, however, the problem was not an unwillingness to consider my unhappiness per se—I did so ad nauseam in poems and diary entries, and during hours spent poring over song lyrics. I just didn't care to do so under the supervision of an adult who couldn't possibly, I thought, understand the depths and nuances of my unhappiness. When, during my senior year, I finally worked up the nerve to discuss medication with my parents, and then to request a Prozac prescription from my pediatrician, I saw medication as a means of liberation. Undoubtedly I did have issues I was not only unwilling to discuss in therapy, but unwilling to admit to myself—and perhaps taking medication was a way of dodging those issues. But Prozac afforded me a level of privacy and dignity that at the time I desperately needed. It also seemed to absolve me of fault: just as the ads on TV said, I had a chemical imbalance that needed medication to be righted.

To judge from the academic literature and parenting books, few adults during the 1990s and even into the millennium were thinking about these questions of autonomy and control with regard to children's psychiatric treatment. Psychiatrists seem to have been caught up in the

general enthusiasm over the new biological psychiatry, while anthropologists and other social scientists studied adults' interpretation of taking medication, not children's. The parenting books, naturally, took
the parents' point of view, explaining how to help kids "manage" their
medication.

Medication management, in fact, had become the new norm for
treatment, as overworked pediatricians prescribed more psychotropics,
and psychiatrists switched to short psychopharmacology consultations.
What doctors were not spending much time doing was talking to children about how they felt about their medication, what some have called
"the psychology of psychopharmacology." A new model of bifurcated
treatment became the norm during the '90s, in part because of the rise
of biological psychiatry, and in part because of financial constraints
imposed by insurance companies: the physicians, both psychiatrists
and general practitioners, handled the meds, while psychologists, social
workers, and other counselors and therapists, plus a dwindling number
of psychoanalysts and psychodynamically minded psychiatrists, mined
children's relationships, behaviors, and moods. With regard to ADHD,
by far the most common disorder, it was sometimes suggested that
counseling would be required for children. The *St. Petersburg Times*
described these children in 1990 as "staggering under twin burdens
of teacher disapproval and parental disappointment."[14] But the possibility of counseling children specifically about their attitudes toward
their medication was rarely discussed either in the psychiatric literature
or the popular media. The prevailing view was that meds provided a
quick fix.

That is not to say that clinicians and researchers weren't concerned
about the potential psychological fallout from taking psychiatric drugs.
They worried that taking medication from a young age would encourage children to attribute ordinary and quite justified emotions to the
drug, a situation that a number of child psychiatrists who have treated
children with medications from the 1990s onward told me they wit-
nessed repeatedly. Psychiatrist David Mintz of Austen Riggs, a long-
term treatment facility in western Massachusetts oriented toward
psychotherapy, works with treatment-resistant patients typically fun-

neled into the mental health system at a young age. "A healthier person thinks, 'Well what does this mean and what should I do with this?'" he explains. "'Does my guilt mean I shouldn't ever do this thing again? Does my anger mean I have to confront somebody?'" But some young people who have spent their formative years taking medication, he has observed, "end up thinking of their feelings not as guides, but simply as symptoms." Debra Emmite, a child and adolescent psychiatrist in Houston, also thinks that medication, and the symptom-based model of biological psychiatry that goes along with it, can cause kids to doubt the authenticity of their emotions. She has noticed particular problems among bipolar teenagers, who are at an age when mood swings are common but who are also contending with the cycling between the highs of mania and lows of depression. "Sometimes they don't know what's a realistic healthy response to a situation versus [whether] they're going up or they're going down," she said.

Other psychiatrists noted that they thought older kids and teens were more likely to look for outside causes, as opposed to inner ones, because they're in a period of development when peer relationships are paramount. A few people I interviewed, including Elizabeth, seemed to have subscribed to that view as teenagers. Adam, the young man from Indiana who suffered a deep and lasting depression over a seventh grade breakup around the time his brother was diagnosed with schizophrenia, described how clearly he viewed the impetus for his unhappiness: he'd lost the love of his young life. And he was skeptical throughout his treatment with the antidepressant Effexor, not understanding "how a pill could affect something so fundamentally intertwined with your soul as your emotions."

Some of the earlier studies concerning the psychological effects of meds concentrated on the ways in which children on stimulants either took ownership, or failed to take ownership, of their success and failures, and how that influenced their attitudes toward their medication. As early as the 1970s concerns surfaced in the research literature that children might become psychologically dependent on stimulants.[15] "As most children mature, their competencies increase, and their successes tend to be attributable more and more to their developing skills, while failures are blamed on lack of effort," the developmental psychologist Carol Whalen wrote in 1983, noting the "risk that diagnosis and medication may interfere with this normal developmental process." She added, of her own experiences treating kids:

> We have heard children credit their pills when they complete their schoolwork, are kind to their pets, clean their rooms, and get invited to parties. They report that the medication prevents them from acting crazy, picking fights, getting kicked out of school, spending all of their money in a single day, and killing frogs! Analogously, forgetting to take medication is blamed for poor grades, temper tantrums, rule infractions, social squabbles, breaking or burying other people's toys, and even rolling toilet paper down the stairs while parents are entertaining![16]

Lawrence Diller, a behavioral pediatrician in the San Francisco Bay Area, raised concerns in his popular 1998 book, *Running on Ritalin*, that children who took stimulants to focus and control their impulses and behavior might become dependent on the drug-induced feeling of security. The phenomenon is especially likely to occur, Diller cautioned in an article in a bioethics journal the following year, when parents and teachers ask, as Paul's foster parents and therapists did, whenever a kid misbehaves, "Did you take your pill today?" That question, Diller writes, "expresses an underlying message to the child about the drug's important contribution to performance and behavior, and, ultimately, this message may undermine the child's confidence."[17]

This concern is probably less relevant for antidepressants, whose effects are only evident after a number of weeks, than it is for short-acting drugs, such as stimulants or some antipsychotics, whose effects, or lack thereof, are immediately apparent. Further, as Diller points out, stimulants are often taken on an as-needed basis—to study for a big exam, say, or to ensure good behavior for a family get-together—thus reinforcing the child's sense that he lacks self-control. Regardless, I think the focus on children's fragile egos fails to give kids enough credit for the creative ways in which they can choose to play with, subvert, or reinterpret the role of "the medicated kid." Even children who feel forced to take medication don't necessarily accept adults' vision of who they are. As the next chapter will explore in more depth, several studies of ADHD from the early '90s demonstrated, for example, that even kids who said the medication helped them fiercely insisted that they—and not the medication—were responsible for how they acted.

Paul, ages nine to ten
FORT LAUDERDALE, FLORIDA / 1997–1998
Whereas Claire embraced her newfound role as a poster child for childhood depression treatment, Paul took his medications because everyone—the foster-care workers, his foster parents, his doctors—told him he had to. And while Elizabeth mostly wanted her parents and school to leave her alone, Paul used his reputation as a "difficult child" who needed meds to wield a little power in a system where he otherwise had none.

When Paul misbehaved or moved to a new foster-care placement, his caseworkers would send him to a psychiatrist to see whether his meds needed adjusting. Paul also received therapy, but he often felt manipulated into saying what he thought the therapists wanted him to say. When asked why he got into a fight at school, for example, Paul would explain that a kid was teasing him for not having parents. The therapist would say something like, "No, Paul, that's not true. You know that's not true. The reason you got into a fight is because you have anger issues. Maybe you didn't take your meds today?" Although his therapists and psychiatrists maintained that Paul wasn't in control of his behavior, he always felt that he made deliberate and reasonable choices to act the way he did. Acting out was a public performance, and he liked to think he knew what he was doing.

Other times, when Paul misbehaved, the psychiatrist would prescribe a higher dosage of medication. Or at least that's how it seemed. No matter how often they altered the dose, Paul never noticed feeling any different. After a while, Paul started giving the grown-ups the explanation they wanted, not because he believed it, but because the idea that he needed meds to control his anger provided a convenient excuse for his behavioral problems. If he was mouthing off in school, he'd tell the teacher, "I didn't take my meds today." Or if he'd behaved badly at home, he'd tell his therapist that his foster parents had been forgetting to give him his pills (sometimes it was true).

Paul's life changed at the age of nine when he finally landed in a foster home he liked. His new foster parents, Dan and Nora, had a nice house and two friendly dogs in a well-kept residential development near a park where Paul loved to go rollerblading. Dan, a firefighter, was strict, but Nora, who didn't work and was always home when Paul got back from school, was more of a softie. At first, Paul acted out a lot, almost to test them, he later concluded. He figured they'd probably send him away, as the other fed-up foster parents had. But they stuck with him.

At school, he continued to play the role of the tough street kid, which impressed his suburban classmates. Maybe because of his initial disobedience at home, or because of his continuing aggression at school, his psychiatrist prescribed a new medication in addition to the Ritalin—an antiseizure drug called Tegretol. Drugs like Tegretol had originally been used in the 1960s and 1970s as anticonvulsant medications to treat epilepsy, but by the 1990s doctors were expanding their use as "mood stabilizers" to curb violent and aggressive behavior in children with ADHD, conduct disorder, oppositional defiant disorder, bipolar disorder, and other such diagnoses proliferating at the time to describe "problem kids." Rates of use, though constituting less than 1 percent of the general youth population, nearly doubled between 1994 and 2003, according to a survey of an HMO in California. One study of children enrolled in a mid-Atlantic state's Medicaid program in the year 2000 found that 81 percent received an anticonvulsant for an emotional or behavioral diagnosis, as opposed to just 19 percent for a seizure disorder. Boys were twice as likely to receive the drugs for psychiatric reasons as girls, as were children with Medicaid compared to those with private insurance.[18]

Whatever Paul's emotional or behavioral diagnosis was, however, he wasn't informed. He just figured this was another drug to try to make him behave. He didn't feel any different taking the Tegretol, just as he didn't feel any different taking Ritalin. When he began behaving better, he attributed it to his own deliberate decision making. He'd proved himself to classmates at his new school, which meant he didn't need to beat up the other kids as much, and Dan and Nora had proved they loved him, so he didn't need to act out at home to test them (although he still resisted when Dan got too strict for his liking). Nora's approach suited him better. When he came home from school and told her he'd had a bad day, she'd give him cookies and milk and rub his back and wipe his runny nose with a tissue and tell him it was okay. Most of the time, though, Paul liked his school a lot—his new friends from the neighborhood went there, and he adored his teacher, who gave him lots of hugs and brought in treats. In this environment, he was less tempted to act out, and didn't find it as hard to focus in class. Also, for the first time, he began to care about getting good grades. Nora would make her special chicken wings when he got an A. When Paul got one B on his report card, he felt like he'd let Dan and Nora down. Paul didn't attribute any of this to his new medication. He credited it to the fact that for the first time, he was getting love and positive reinforcement, rather than neglect or punishment. And when the other foster kid who had been staying with them left, and Paul had a room—and Dan and Nora—all to himself, he got all the more attention.

Dan and Nora didn't have kids of their own, but they talked a lot about wanting to adopt children. Not understanding that he was staying with them under a so-called therapeutic foster-care arrangement that was strictly temporary, Paul desperately hoped they'd adopt him. Instead, shortly after his tenth birthday, Dan and Nora explained that they were going to adopt two other kids around his age, a brother and sister Paul knew from one of the group homes he'd lived in a few years earlier. Paul was crushed. He thought he'd behaved very well all year long—his psychiatrist, whom he saw once a month, hadn't upped his dosage of either medication in a long time, and Dan and Nora sometimes didn't even seem to notice when they forgot to give Paul his meds. But if they wanted to adopt other kids instead of him, maybe he hadn't been as well behaved as he thought.

The children had lived with Dan and Nora before, which made it even more difficult for Paul to understand why he was temporary, while they would be Dan and Nora's children forever. When they moved in,

Paul felt Dan and Nora change, become less affectionate. On weekends, they would drop him off at the community center and take the other kids on "bonding" excursions. The boy lorded this over Paul. When they were watching TV and Paul would try to change the channel, the boy would say, "These are my parents, and this is my house, and I get to watch the channel *I* want." Hurt and jealous, Paul would beat him up.

One weekend, Dan and Nora were preparing to take the other two kids away for some bonding, intending to leave Paul in a short-term respite home. A little while before it was time to leave, Paul saw his medication bottles lined up on the kitchen counter. Suddenly, it occurred to him that maybe if he took a whole bunch of pills at once, they would fix him for good, and then Dan and Nora would want to adopt him. He swallowed the contents of both bottles and then got in the car with Dan, Nora, and the other kids.

The lady at the respite home had a nice condo with a pool, which cheered him up some, as did the hamburgers she made him for lunch. As Paul was eating, he noticed the walls and doorknobs moving. He asked what was going on. "The doorknob's not moving by itself," the woman said. "Are you okay?" She told him to go lie down on the couch, but it looked like there were two or three couches lined up next to each other. The next thing Paul knew, he woke up in the hospital. The nurses told him he had almost died.

Paul wasn't chastened. He usually enjoyed being in the hospital, because he liked being fussed over. Sometimes, he had even misbehaved on purpose so he'd be sent to the hospital for a three-day cooling-off period. Sure enough, the staff catered to him again this time—he got a Sega Genesis, the newest and coolest video game system, delivered right to his room, and the late-night cook brought him midnight snacks. Pretty soon, he felt like his usual hyperactive self, running up and down the hallways of the hospital as if it were his playground, even bursting in during an operation. He got to stay two weeks, while the doctors made sure he was okay from the overdose and then started him on a new medication in addition to the Ritalin. Paul didn't mind—the Tegretol tasted like gross bubble gum. He was glad to be rid of it.

But once he got back to Dan and Nora's, things were no better. The police were looking into how he had overdosed, suspecting that the lady at the respite home had given him all those pills at once. There was a big meeting at the foster-care office with Paul, Dan and Nora, his caseworkers, therapist, psychiatrist, and a bunch of other adults. Despite the scrutiny, Paul never admitted he'd taken all those pills himself; he didn't really understand why it was so serious, and didn't make the connection between the overdose and having almost died. Instead, he let everyone conclude that perhaps the lady at the respite home had just messed up his dosage by mistake.

Paul wasn't sure yet what to think about his medication, but he did know that taking all those pills hadn't, as he'd hoped, morphed him into a good kid, a kid who did well in school and made his foster parents proud. He'd been trying to play that role all year, but he realized he'd failed when Dan and Nora told him they were going to adopt two other kids. Now, he'd failed again. Dan and Nora were relieved he was okay, of course, but it wasn't as though they had rushed into his hospital room to tell him tearfully that they'd been wrong and that they intended to adopt him on the spot. If anything, Paul thought, the episode had convinced them that he was trouble—that they'd been right all along not to choose him as their son.

Paul made one last-ditch effort to change their minds. Nora was always the more nurturing of the two, so he approached her. "Nora, is there a way I can stay? I promise I'll call you Mom. I promise I'll be a good kid."

Nora looked surprised. "You don't have to call me Mom," she told him. "But don't worry—you're going to be happy the next place you go."

CHAPTER 3

School Interventions

*About five years ago, teachers heard the welcome news
that small doses of amphetamines and other psychoactive drugs
could turn hyperactive children into willing learners.
As a result, an estimated 300,000 children now are taking these drugs
—and many of them should not be.*

— *Time* MAGAZINE, 1973

By the time children's stimulant prescriptions began to spike in the late
1980s, the issues of academic achievement, rowdy schoolchildren, and
Ritalin were already inextricably linked in the public imagination. Fifteen years earlier, Congress had conducted hearings after reports that
15 percent of children in Omaha public schools were taking stimulants
to control hyperactivity. Members of the congressional subcommittee
warned that the drugs were being used to control "bored but bright"
schoolchildren, and anecdotal reports of teachers pressuring parents
to medicate their unruly kids appeared in the media.[1] A backlash en-
sued, with the number of stimulant prescriptions dipping and many
parents embracing the popular Feingold diet plan, which promised to
control kids' behavior by eliminating artificial colors, flavors, and certain preservatives. When prescribing picked up again in the late 1980s,
schools came to the fore of the debate. A rash of lawsuits, many led by
the antipsychiatry Church of Scientology, charged school districts with

pressuring parents to medicate their children. Oprah, Phil Donahue, and other talk show hosts devoted shows to the controversy, and a slew of headlines made the inevitable connection: " 'R' Is for Ritalin," "Ritalin: Education's Fix-It Drug?" "Hyperactivity 'Miracle Drug' Comes under Heavy Fire." "Faced with rambunctious, contrary, or unfocused children," the education magazine *Phi Delta Kappan* asked in 1989, "are schools leaping to the conclusion that drugs can solve the problem? Is the education system neglecting to try alternative approaches that might work for youngsters who are not easily managed—who have difficulty, as education jargon would have it, 'staying on task?' "[2]

It was a natural question to ask—so natural, in fact, that a grade schooler might wonder as much herself. I entered first grade in 1989, the same year the *Phi Delta Kappan* article came out, and rather quickly came to some similar conclusions. The few classmates who traipsed off every day around noon to the school nurse's office for the pill to "help them behave" were, I soon discerned, the same children who tended to talk during class, tip back perilously in their chairs, poke their desk mates with pencils, and pick fights during recess. I didn't know what kind of medicine they took, but the reasons for its administration were utterly clear to me: some kids just couldn't—or wouldn't—behave. That much was evident from all the time my elementary school classes spent standing in line, waiting to go to lunch, gym, or recess: the rule was that the line couldn't go anywhere until everyone was perfectly quiet. Inevitably, that took some time to achieve and was significantly delayed by the usual suspects. I didn't think about it then, but I wonder now if the line would ever have moved, but for their meds.

The fact is, despite pronouncements about educating young minds, a significant portion of elementary school, and even of middle and high school, is spent simply trying to get everyone to quiet down and listen to the teacher. My elementary school, in a liberal college town, paid lip service to the educational vogue of different learning styles, and in fact placed a significant emphasis on creative and collaborative projects. But like other schools, it demanded a certain level of order and conformity to fulfill its basic mission of efficiently educating as many children as possible. The kids who were not severely disabled but who consistently interfered with those attempts at order were naturally going to attract the most attention from both teachers and classmates. That had been the case from time immemorial; the difference by the late 1980s and early 1990s was that many of the troublemakers were taking stimulant medications like Ritalin, or soon would be.

As more medications became available to manage distracting and aggressive behavior, schools increasingly encouraged, even pressured, parents or guardians to medicate disruptive kids. Federal and state special education law required children with certain defined disorders that impaired learning to be individually accommodated, but schools often saw meds as a way to avoid providing these expensive special services. Strapped for resources, they mostly did not provide the kind of comprehensive support system necessary to help kids deal with the psychological and logistical complexities that result from being on psychotropic drugs.

To further complicate the situation, kids who internalized their problems and didn't impose them on the class often slipped under the radar; in contrast to peers who had full-scale, debilitating impairments, such as severe autism or mental retardation, they were relatively high-functioning. A child might have such severe anxiety that some days she was simply unable to go to school, or such severe compulsions that she couldn't concentrate on what the teacher was saying. Some of these kids received medications that worked sufficiently to resolve their symptoms and help them function. But others received medications that didn't work at all, or that resolved some symptoms but not others, and these children didn't always receive the kind of support or accommodations they needed in order to perform up to their full potential. A student who sat listlessly in his seat and turned in mediocre homework might be severely depressed or distracted by obsessive thoughts, but he stood out less than the hyperactive ADHD kid who disrupted class and constantly lost his homework, the child with oppositional defiant disorder who confronted authority figures at every turn, or the teenager with conduct disorder who beat up classmates and destroyed school property. Since teachers and staff often lacked the knowledge or resources to identify and help kids with psychological problems of all sorts, it was—and, as journalist Judith Warner's book *We've Got Issues: Children and Parents in the Age of Medication* convincingly demonstrates, still is—largely up to their parents to be proactive and seek the necessary accommodations, a process that requires considerable time, know-how, and resources.[3] Children who did not or could not articulate or demonstrate their problems, or whose parents or guardians were unable or unwilling to intervene, continued to suffer.

As a result, the issues of unruly kids with disruptive behavior disorders, ADHD in particular, dominated the conversation about medication and learning in the 1990s. ADHD was not only the most commonly diagnosed disorder, and stimulants such as Ritalin the most commonly prescribed class of medications, but a high percentage of children with behavior disorders are also diagnosed with a "specific learning disorder" in a particular subject area, or with a disorder, for example, affecting written expression or auditory processing. The exact prevalence of comorbidity between learning disabilities and behavior disorders like ADHD, conduct disorder, and oppositional defiant disorder ranges widely between studies, but the preeminent ADHD researcher Russell Barkley estimated in 1994 that between 25 and 50 percent of children with ADHD had a learning disability.[4] Although numerous studies had shown stimulants to be effective for improving focus and reducing hyperactivity, the evidence did not support the drugs' use to treat specific learning disabilities. Prevailing expert opinion by the 1990s held that these learning problems required remedial or other supplemental services at school, while ADHD symptoms could improve as a result of both medication and other interventions, including accommodations such as allowing extra time on tests and placing easily distracted students in the front row to help them concentrate. In my elementary school, I noticed that the children who took pills from the nurse also went to the "resource room" for "special help" at certain times during the day. Looking back, I suspect that not all of my medicated classmates in fact received special education services, but at the time it was easy to assume as much, especially since most of the children I knew who took behavioral medications and got extra academic help were also periodically sent to this same "resource room" to cool off when they were uncontrollably loud, aggressive, or defiant. In my mind, it all blended together—the noontime journeys to the nurse for medication, the acting out, and the extra help—all markers of some vague constellation of problems that was at once obvious and hard to define.

On the surface, then, the issues about schools and medication seemed clear-cut, but the deeper researchers and commentators delved, the murkier and more complex they turned out to be. In the realm of rhetoric and public debate, adults argued about whether stimulants were chemical babysitters used instead of deserved accommodations for legitimate disabilities. In 2000, in something of a replay of its investigation from the early '70s, Congress again held hearings to investigate, among other issues, whether schools were unduly pressuring parents to medicate rowdy students, or whether medication was a proven and legitimate means of helping bright but distracted children achieve their potential. Although coverage of the hearings tended to frame the issue in such absolute terms, for the children who actually took medication—not to mention their parents—the relationship between pharmaceutical treatment and learning was anything but simple. It begged all kinds of questions about what a school owed a child with behavioral or emotional troubles and a prescription.

The fact was that stimulants, the drugs most closely tied to academic achievement, the best studied, and the most commonly prescribed of the psychotropic medications, did not reliably create either overachieving super-pupils or conformist automatons. Schools did not either lavish personalized educations on children or ignore them and let the pills drug pupils into submission. Nor was a prescription for a stimulant or any other medication an automatic pass to special services at school. Rather, an intricate and ever-shifting dance took shape between academic achievement, school accommodations, and psychotropic drugs. It was, however, a dance little discussed outside of professional, educational, and mental health circles.

Paul, ages five to eleven
FORT LAUDERDALE, FLORIDA / 1993–2000
A school's involvement in a child's psychiatric treatment could range from nonexistent—not even knowing the child was receiving treat-

ment—to a full array of adjunctive accommodations meant to supplement the effects of the medication or fill in gaps where medication was not effective. Paul was one child who got a full raft of such services, including, for much of elementary school starting in the first or second grade, a slot in specialized behavioral schools. In theory the various adults in Paul's life—his psychiatrists, therapists, foster parents, case manager and mental health case manager, teachers and school psychologists—were supposed to be exchanging information about his treatment, behavior, and academic performance in order to work out an integrated treatment plan. But it's not evident that they clearly or accurately communicated with one another. Ensconced from an early age in this network of systems, all of them providing or purporting to provide various services pertaining to his behavior and emotional health, Paul himself made little distinction among them. He saw school accommodations as just one more result of his acting out, like his medication, or like his frequently changing home placements.

From the time Paul started school, he'd been a troublemaker, beating up other kids when they said or did something that upset him. When he was in a good mood he would fool around in class and make everyone laugh, but that could also be disruptive. Adults didn't talk about his medication—either the Ritalin he was first prescribed or Tegretol, the mood stabilizer he received a little later—in terms of helping him learn or get better grades. The way Paul understood it, the drugs were strictly to calm him down and prevent him from making trouble. Perhaps as a result, he didn't think a whole lot about the arrangements schools made to help him learn. Mostly he just noticed when he was segregated in a separate class, or even in a separate school, with other disruptive kids. Although he had an individualized education plan (IEP) explicitly granting him access to certain special education services under federal law, Paul didn't even know what an IEP was until high school. When he did get individualized learning help or assessments, he thought his teachers wanted to spend extra time with him because they liked him. Lacking parental affection, he welcomed any attention, even being sent to the "ice room" because he threw a desk at a teacher or punched another kid.

While some critics of special education complained that it enabled savvy, well-connected, wealthy parents to secure disproportionate advantages for their kids, others contended that by the 1990s special ed had become merely a place to "warehouse" the most troubled and worst-performing students, especially poor or minority children like Paul, in separate classes with lower standards. Indeed, although many states implemented standardized competency testing in the 1980s and 1990s, there was wide variation among states in their requirements for special education students. In high school, for example, Paul's IEP exempted him from the Florida state tests required for graduation.

As a middle schooler, Paul would come to yearn to attend a mainstream school, but during elementary school, at least, he didn't feel warehoused in behavioral programs. He didn't particularly mind that during the time he was placed with Dan and Nora he had to repeat third grade in order to be admitted to a well-respected behavioral program. Most of the time, he appreciated the lack of homework, the untimed tests, and the chance to earn rewards for good behavior. And, as he did with his foster-care placements, he took a particular pleasure in manipulating people and situations to his advantage. He and his best friend, Matt, whom he met in third grade while living at Dan and Nora's house, enjoyed working the system. Matt also took Ritalin, and the boys once engineered a memorable coup when Paul, on his way back from the nurse for meds, and Matt, on his way there, teamed up while unsupervised to pick a fight with another kid. As usual, Matt did the trash talking to get the kid mad, and Paul did the beating up.

This system didn't last, though. Paul loved the school he attended while living with Dan and Nora and was crushed when, shortly after his reluctant departure from their house, he was expelled for fighting. After that, Paul was bounced in rapid succession from one home placement to another, acting out in hopes of being transferred someplace better, always hoping to find another place as good as Dan and Nora's. And, as before, each new foster home occasioned a new school, which added to the disruption and discontinuity of his life. At some point, around Paul's fifth grade year, the foster system decided he should be placed in a behavioral school that he could attend regardless of where he lived in order to minimize disruptions and allow him, in light of his very troubling behaviors, a full range of services.

"Alternative schools" like the one Paul was assigned to were proliferating in the 1990s, partly as a result of the school choice and charter
school movements, and partly as a result of growing fears about school
violence and the widely implemented "zero tolerance policies" for
crime, drugs, and violent behavior. Alternative schools had sprung up
across the country in the 1960s and 1970s as part of an overall school reform movement that emphasized more creative, less restrictive learning
environments. The movement waned toward the end of the 1970s—a
1981 *New York Times* article asked "Whatever Happened to Alternative
Schools?"[5]—but revived again by the end of the 1980s as public schools
began to emphasize school choice, expanding their magnet school programs and also providing alternative learning centers for kids deemed
to be at risk, marginal, or disadvantaged. On occasion, these alternative
schools attracted criticism for lax educational standards. A 2000 inves-
tigative article in the *Oregonian*, Portland's well-respected daily paper,
found that alternative schools across the state operated with little over-
sight, poor facilities, and bare-bones curricula, generally acting "more
as a sieve than as a safety net."[6]

Paul, though, liked his behavioral school. Among the services he
received were twice-weekly one-on-one therapy sessions with a school
psychologist, in addition to regular therapy and medication management visits outside of school. In contrast to his out-of-school therapy,
where he frequently felt that the counselors put words in his mouth, Paul
enjoyed his school sessions. He got to miss class, and he relished getting
a chance to ask the psychologist questions pertaining to sex, given that
other adults in his life tended to ignore such prurient inquiries. At the
school, medication was commonplace, doled out in little cups to much
of the class. So was taking "the short bus" for special education kids,
something that had gotten Paul teased at the school he attended while
at Dan and Nora's. (Paul had put a stop to the teasing with his usual
strategy of beating up anyone who challenged him.) Here, neither his
medication nor his accommodations troubled him intensely. It would
be another year or two before he'd get seriously interested in girls, and
then, wanting to appear as cool and attractive as possible, he would want
to leave the special schools—and his medication—behind.

• • •

To a great extent, how children felt about the school's involvement in their psychiatric problems depended on how visible their disorder was, and whether they considered treatment a public or a private matter. For Paul the boundaries between public and private weren't so clear because most of his time was spent in an institutional context. So the fact that he took medications during school, saw a therapist there, and also got accommodations was unremarkable. But other children I interviewed took these boundaries between public and private more seriously. Some liked the assistance they received in school because, like Paul, they felt that any attention was good attention. Some appreciated the chance to vent to sympathetic guidance counselors or school psychologists. The majority of the young people with whom I spoke, however, considered their mental health treatment a private matter, something they wanted to keep separate from school. Short-acting stimulants like regular-release Ritalin made them more visible at school because they had to go to the nurse for a midday dose, but as more long-acting formulations came on the market in the late 1990s and after, that proved less of a problem. As for accommodations, most didn't consider such arrangements necessary, so long as their medication worked well; in fact, many of them welcomed the medication because it enabled them to avoid being treated differently in school. "I didn't want to be held back because people feel sorry for me," said one young man, Caleb, who had been diagnosed and medicated for severe depression and post-traumatic stress disorder (PTSD) when he was thirteen. Pep rallies, with their noise and jostling, triggered flashbacks to the severe bullying that had precipitated his PTSD, but attendance was required and he would never have considered asking special permission to be excused. He didn't want his classmates to wonder where he was. "Eventually they might figure out that I had depression," he said. "And I [didn't] want them to treat me any different."

Though I didn't receive medication until my senior year in high school, I could identify with that logic. Indeed, long before I actually got a prescription, the treatment appealed to me in part because I didn't care to discuss my problems with adults. I don't think I even knew whether my high school had a therapist. It did have guidance counselors, but they seemed to exist to deal with the "problem kids"—the ones who got pregnant in eighth grade and skipped class to go smoke in the bathroom. Medication was also appealing because it allowed me to maintain my public image as a self-motivated, high achiever. During my middle school scoliosis treatment I cringed at the few accommodations my parents arranged, such as having me leave gym class early so my best friend could help me rush back into my brace before my classmates saw. By comparison, medication seemed marvelously invisible.

My peers and I attended school at a time when educators were becoming increasingly involved in more aspects of children's lives. As the historian Steven Mintz recounts in his history of American childhood, *Huck's Raft*, schools in the 1990s implemented a host of measures, including zero-tolerance policies for alcohol and drugs, uniforms, and backpack and locker searches, that reflected larger cultural concerns over school violence and crime, and a perceived erosion of parental authority. These measures intensified the sense that children's private lives weren't their own, which, I think, made me and many of my peers guard our private turmoil all the more closely.[7]

Even while encroaching on students' privacy, schools failed to resolve the ongoing question of how involved they should be in their pupils' emotional lives. From the 1970s on there was a move to take children's overall well-being into account as an important factor in shaping their academic commitment and achievement. More schools added psychologists, social workers, and even psychiatrists to their staffs, or kept them on as official liaisons. In the early 1990s, as the number of children taking psychotropic drugs surged, the school psychology profession even floated the idea of obtaining special dispensation to prescribe and monitor medications, as a way of better integrating children's out-of-school treatment with the services they received in school. The larger movement to give prescribing privileges to psychologists progressed slowly, with New Mexico, the first state to grant licensed psychologists with doctoral-level degrees prescribing authority, not enacting such a law until 2002, and only a few more doing so since.[8] In practice, however, school mental health personnel found their roles more and more circumscribed as the decade progressed. Budget cuts forced psychologists and social workers to circulate within the school system, often hopping among several schools daily. As the number of children and families seeking accommodations soared, the school support staff became overwhelmed, conducting learning assessments to fulfill state and federal special education requirements. Teachers and guidance counselors were left to identify, often on an ad hoc basis, "troubled children" who might need treatment, while school nurses typically dealt with the more prosaic task of monitoring and dispensing medications that needed to be taken during the school day. Integrating children's existing, outside mental health treatment with their lives at school in any comprehensive way was usually beyond schools' limited resources. Even at small, elite schools like the one Elizabeth attended in Washington, DC, students could easily slip, or even actively wiggle, through the cracks.

Elizabeth, ages fourteen to eighteen
WASHINGTON, DC, SUBURBS / 1995–1999

After Elizabeth was diagnosed with ADHD and depression at the beginning of ninth grade and prescribed Ritalin and Prozac, she started reading everything she could find on ADHD, trying to understand why she seemed to be performing "below her potential" in school. She knew from various aptitude tests she'd taken, including the entrance examination for her elite private school, that she scored in the top percentile for most measures of ability, even though her school performance was uneven. Previously, she'd attributed her academic failures to lack of effort. But books, such as the recent best seller *Driven to Distraction*, mentioned various accommodations that could help even if children were already taking stimulants.

Liz had undergone psychological testing a couple of years earlier, at the urging of the family therapist, who had a child with ADHD. The testing found that she was extraordinarily bright, but that she had memory, attention, and writing problems. Liz knew her mother had given the results of the testing to her school in an attempt to secure some accommodations, but when, inspired by her reading, she inquired whether her mother had followed up with the school, her mom explained that the law required only public schools, not private institutions, to provide accommodations. Liz knew from her reading, however, that her mother was wrong. The federal Americans with Disabilities Act of 1990 had extended existing protections, which had previously applied only to institutions receiving public funding, to private schools. That meant that her school needed to provide "reasonable accommodations" to any student who could demonstrate a "physical or mental disability that substantially interferes with one or more major life activities."[9] What she didn't know was whether her school received federal funds. However, one thing she knew for sure was that her school provided accommodations to many students already.

Liz recounted all of this to her parents, to no avail. Their lack of interest infuriated her, not least because her father was a lawyer at a powerful and prestigious DC law firm. She had heard him stridently argue on her older sister's behalf and knew that when he wanted to, he could get things done. (She also knew, by this point, that her father was a recovering alcoholic who'd been in and out of sobriety for years.) Of course her parents had their own worries, caught up as they were in marital strife. They may also have figured that her prescription for stimulants ought to resolve any academic problems she had. But to Liz, who didn't notice any dramatic effects from the stimulants anyway, her parents' lack of interest in learning more about ADHD and securing school accommodations symbolized the many ways they had been absent and unsupportive ever since their marital problems had begun some unknown number of years earlier. Their attitude all along had been, "We just want you to do your best, and we know you're capable of getting straight A's if you just do your homework." They didn't seem to understand that she *was* trying, but that even with medication, her disorder was keeping her back.

Whether as a result of the Ritalin and Prozac or for other reasons, Liz's grades improved to As and Bs during ninth and tenth grade. But that merely raised her parents' expectations. In eighth grade, they had just been relieved that she didn't fail out of school; now they *really* expected her to get straight A's. One day in tenth grade, her mother brought up her grades yet again. "Elizabeth," her mom said, "you don't do your homework. That doesn't have anything to do with ADHD." Liz's head just about exploded: kids with ADHD, she wanted to scream, don't do their homework because they have trouble getting organized and focusing. How could her mom not process that? Even as she resented her mother's words, though, she identified with her parents' assessment that she wasn't, in fact, performing as well as she could have, despite the boost she received from the medication. At heart, she was a perfectionist.

In addition to reading parent-advice books on ADHD, Liz read everything she could find in popular publications such as the *New York Times* and *Newsweek*. She was familiar with and angered by the litany of criticisms about ADHD and medication. For one thing, people often dismissed ADHD as just "boys being boys," and assumed that they'd outgrow it. But Liz knew better. Many doctors thought the condition had long been underdiagnosed in kids like her—girls (and boys) who were easily distracted, but not hyperactive or disruptive.

The hypothesis that overburdened schools pushed medication on kids as a quick fix didn't resonate with her personal experience, either. Liz's small, private school was brimming with resources and expertise, and prided itself on close contact with both students and parents. Two school therapists had approached her individually—one in eighth grade before she went on medication, and the other in ninth, after she had begun taking it—to see if she wanted to talk, but she had been too shy and mortified to take advantage of the offers. When she was especially depressed and floundering in eighth grade, a teacher gave her a tape of soothing ocean sounds and other relaxation music and invited Liz to talk to her if she ever needed help. Even if the school wasn't taking the initiative to provide academic accommodations, Liz knew the administrators couldn't be adamantly opposed. By ninth or tenth grade, she was aware of classmates, including those who took medication for ADHD, receiving extra time on tests and other arrangements, and knew there even a special guidance counselor for kids with disabilities. The school was certainly equipped to help kids like her, Liz thought. Her parents just weren't holding up their end.

The irony was that the media made it sound as if parents like hers—wealthy, white, well-educated—were cannily seeking advantages for their kids at every turn by securing diagnoses and medications for ADHD, and then lobbying for special accommodations to boot. As Liz saw it, her parents' involvement was frustratingly limited to nagging her about her grades and, in her mother's case, occasionally urging her to see a therapist in addition to taking medication. Liz felt unable to advocate for herself. For a while toward the end of high school, she considered deliberately getting into trouble, knowing that the school would punish her by replacing her free period with a study hall, which would force her to do her homework in a supervised environment. But she couldn't quite bring herself to act out on purpose, nor to approach the dean of students and request a study hall outright.

Complicating everything was the reality that neither Ritalin nor Prozac had managed to turn her into a superfocused whiz kid, especially compared to her very bright and highly motivated classmates. With regard to Ritalin specifically, she was willing to give it a stab insofar as it did what the doctor said it was supposed to do for her academically. There were still times, though, when she wondered if her parents were right. Even if she did have ADHD, she wasn't sure the diagnosis was sufficient to explain why she consistently underachieved relative to what the standardized tests, neuropsychological testing, and other measures indicated she should be capable of doing.

When it came time to take the SATs, she could have applied for special provisions, such as extra time, based on her ADHD. Such accommodations had been available since the early 1980s. Between 1990 and 1999, when Liz took the SAT, the percentage of students taking the nonstandard version of the test because of a learning disorder or ADHD, as opposed to physical or other disabilities, increased from 15 percent to 42 percent.[10] In 1999, though, the College Board was still flagging any scores taken under special testing conditions when it sent the results on to colleges. Liz didn't request the extra time, afraid that the admissions officers would question her abilities if she received accommodations—but she did make sure to take her Ritalin the day of the test.

Circumstances like hers were among the most controversial, because they explicitly raised the question of what purpose accommodations served: did they help compensate for low-achieving students' deficits, or did they enable all children with a disability, even if they were extremely bright, to achieve the highest score they could? The year after Liz took the SAT, a California audit of ACT/SAT test takers found that a disproportionate percentage of those receiving accommodations on the tests were white and wealthy, "igniting suspicions," as the *New York Times* put it, "of exaggerated or nonexistent disabilities." Three years later, after a lawsuit, both the SAT and the ACT stopped flagging scores. Since then, the organizations are said to have tightened their standards, to prevent students from gaming the system: students now have to prove they were granted and took advantage of accommodations at school, that their disability limits their ability to take the standard test, and that the requested accommodation fits their disability. Late diagnosis, occurring just before or during high school, is now also considered a red flag, requiring more extensive documentation.[11]

Because taking the test with accommodations was so fraught, Liz balked. It seemed a more public act than simply receiving ADHD-related accommodations from her school. She took the standard test, and despite having failed to study or do any preparation, earned a 1500, just 100 points off a perfect score. A friend she didn't consider as bright scored 10 points higher, which bothered her. She thought about retaking the test, knowing that if she'd studied she almost certainly would have scored higher. But she also knew that even with Ritalin, she wouldn't be able to make herself study enough to make a difference, so a 1500 it was.

Liz was frustrated that her school and her parents didn't work together to get her the academic accommodations she believed she deserved because of her ADHD. She had a strong sense of her own innate intelligence, saw her disorder as keeping her from doing as well academically as she ought to have, and considered Ritalin as a potentially useful but often insufficient tool to remedy her weaknesses. Taking it after school, for example, she was prone to concentrate intently on a video game for hours at a stretch and not get to her homework until late, by which time the drug had worn off. By the time Liz starting taking Ritalin, she was in ninth grade; most kids with ADHD were diagnosed and treated much younger and arguably had more time to develop better study habits with the benefit of the drug.

Some clinicians and researchers worried that pairing academic performance with stimulant treatment could induce a kind of "learned helplessness" in which children came to believe that without the meds they were unable to focus and, therefore, to learn. Such an attitude might prompt them to request an endless string of accommodations and propping-up mechanisms, even at an age when they ought to learn to take responsibility for their behavior and their achievements.

Concerns over learned helplessness provoked a small body of research in the 1980s and 1990s, with mixed results. A series of studies conducted with children in a special summer program for ADHD produced evidence contradicting the theory, finding that those children randomly assigned to receive Ritalin persisted longer on difficult puzzle challenges and solved more puzzles overall than those given a placebo or no medication. Most importantly, the boys who took Ritalin were more likely than those on placebo to attribute their success to their own effort and their failures to external causes, such as the puzzles being hard, or the Ritalin not working, a self-protective, "positive illusory" attitude that most people, except depressed people, exhibit. The researchers speculated that the enabling effects of the medication, rather than the idea of taking a pill, actually helped the children feel empowered and gave them a greater sense of their own abilities.[12]

One intriguing study, interviewing a small group of college students with ADHD about their childhood experiences, found that both the disorder and medication took a toll on the kids' self-image at school. School "taxed their fragile self-esteem," the study's authors wrote, because it was evident to the kids that they had trouble fulfilling basic expectations "to sit still, pay attention, and grasp concepts quickly." Some participants recalled realizing they were different from their classmates as early as first grade. However, diagnosis and medication produced their own problems with stigma and perceived lack of self-sufficiency.[13]

The issue of learned helplessness as a possible result of stimulant treatment also found traction beyond academia. A 1997 column in the *Wall Street Journal* explored the issue through the story of an eight-year-old with ADHD who had been taking Ritalin since age three. The boy's parents had his second grade teacher write progress notes about his behavior each day. The notes said things like, "Tim really, really tries, but he just can't help himself." Other days they said, "Clearly his medication wasn't working well today," sending the message, the column's author wrote, that "either way, the medication or the 'disorder' is responsible; Tim's just along for the ride."[14] Variations on this general argument continue today, with some contending that children learn to rely on medication as a crutch both in school and out, while others argue that medications give children who are used to failure, especially in school and in academic situations, a sense of empowerment.

The debate about learned helplessness is particularly urgent vis-à-vis short-acting stimulant medications prescribed on an as-needed basis, with "medication vacations" during school holidays, for example, requiring parents and kids to constantly assess whether the child needs medication to perform. The same issues potentially arise with other short-acting medications, such as antianxiety drugs or sleeping pills, but these drugs were not—and still aren't—as commonly prescribed to children and teenagers. In the case of a drug one has determined one needs indefinitely, as Claire understood her antidepressants, the issue becomes how to craft a workable, long-term strategy for encouraging learning and academic success. In Claire's mother's opinion, that meant enlisting the school's cooperation, as much as possible, to fill in the gaps where Claire's medication fell short.

Claire, ages eleven to fifteen
HUDSON, OHIO / 1991–1995

Even before her depression, diagnosis, and medication treatment, Claire had been accustomed to her mom's hands-on approach to education. Penny had long been involved with the school, volunteering, fund-raising, and intervening when necessary. In third grade, when two girls—one of them Claire's former friend—began tormenting Claire relentlessly, making Claire so anxious that she refused to attend school,

Penny told the school that if it didn't stop the bullying situation, it would have to send a private tutor to their home. The threat worked. In fourth and fifth grade, Penny made sure Claire's teachers knew she'd been bullied in the past, and secured promises that such a thing wouldn't be tolerated in their classrooms. At the time, Claire was enormously grateful her mom had stepped in, because the only way she knew to respond to the situation had been to curl up under the covers and cry.

In sixth grade, when Claire started middle school, Penny immediately alerted the teachers that Claire had been unable to sleep all summer and seemed to be getting increasingly volatile. When Claire's pediatrician diagnosed her with depression and prescribed a tricyclic antidepressant, Penny apprised Claire's teachers right away. And when the drug seemed only to intensify Claire's mood swings and meltdowns, Penny asked the school for an extra set of books to keep at home in case Claire was too upset to attend. If she stayed home, Claire wasn't allowed to talk on the phone, watch TV, or see her friends after school.

Switching to Prozac in seventh grade alleviated Claire's tantrums, suicide threats, and difficulties focusing, which improved home life for her parents and siblings. However, Claire found herself unable to get through a class period without falling asleep. At the time, she and her parents assumed the drowsiness was a residual symptom of depression; it wasn't until many years later that they realized that the medication might have caused or exacerbated her sleepiness. Whereas Claire's sixth grade arrangements had been ad hoc, this year Penny wanted to make everything official. She had researched federal disabilities law and knew that under a 1973 antidiscrimination statute, section 504 of the Rehabilitation Act, public schools had to accommodate children with any disability that "substantially limits" one or more major life activities. The law listed learning as a major life activity and included emotional or mental illness as a possible qualifying disability.

Penny contended that Claire, having been diagnosed with depression, was still in some ways disabled by her condition despite taking medication. She drew up a list of provisions she demanded from the school, and attached a letter from Claire's psychiatrist. The school granted Claire a so-called 504 plan authorizing the requested accommodations: open-ended deadlines to complete homework assignments, extra time on tests as needed, and unlimited tardiness and absences. Claire also received blanket permission to excuse herself from class and go to the nurse's office or to her guidance counselor should she get too upset to function.

Surveying accommodations for other children she knew, Penny thought Claire's school was unusually responsive to special needs. Yet it occurred to Penny that the school may have been more amenable to Claire's arrangements because the provisions cost nothing and required little extra of the teachers. Compared to the kinds of services parents of more severely disturbed children were seeking at the time— reimbursement for private school tuition when the public schools were allegedly unable to adequately educate the child, for example—Claire's needs were minor.

Moreover, Penny was careful to make clear that she wasn't requesting special arrangements arbitrarily. The provisions in Claire's 504 plan addressed problems that medication didn't adequately treat, and as such, they fit into a well-thought-out, coherent plan of treatment, something resembling, in fact, the kind of comprehensive, "wraparound" care that health policy experts advocate, but which in actuality rarely exists. With Prozac, Claire had markedly improved in certain areas (her meltdowns, her clarity of thought, her organizational skills, her motivation), but like Elizabeth she still got agitated about her homework—math, especially, sent her into a panicked tailspin. Where Elizabeth's anxiety resulted in her simply not completing her homework, though, Claire's accommodations allowed her to simply postpone working until she calmed down. Sometimes she showed up without her assignments, but more often she stayed home to complete whatever work she had been unable to finish the day before. Missing school was better than spending a class period working herself into a frenzy worrying that she didn't understand the material. The unlimited absences and tardiness helped when she needed to make up work, or when she couldn't sleep, since medication had done little for her insomnia and late-night ruminating.

During the first half of seventh grade, Claire was often absent, perhaps two or three days out of every ten, as her mother remembers it. Penny never nagged Claire to attend. She'd say, "I don't know how you're feeling, but if you are too nervous or upset to go to school, that's okay." At one point midway through seventh grade, Claire remarked that wow, she *had* actually been missing an awful lot of school. Penny deadpanned, "Well, that's okay, hon. You don't have to finish seventh grade in one year."

Claire, now twelve and in scornful adolescent mode, couldn't stand such apparent indifference. What *planet* was her mom on that kids just didn't have to go to school when they didn't feel like it? Didn't her mom know that teachers expected seventh graders to be *responsible?* In front of her mother, she didn't back down, but in the following weeks Penny noticed that Claire had fewer absences. She didn't want to be thought of as one of those kids who would try to dodge school out of sheer laziness.

Throughout middle and high school, Claire vacillated between gratitude for the school accommodations and guilt. Feeling sheepish at times, she feared that she was somehow gaming the system. Yet being a depressed kid on medication had become a major part of her identity and image, especially after she made *Claire's Story* in eighth grade and began speaking about her experience at mental health conventions and even to some local and national media. Furthermore, she did consider herself to some extent handicapped by her insomnia, persistent daytime drowsiness, and concentration problems. Often, her parents would go to mental health advocacy events and report back to Claire that they'd met teachers from other schools who said Penny and Fred should be sure to take it easy on her. Both Claire and her parents thought that was amusing. Holding herself to rigorous academic standards, Claire had always been her own harshest critic.

Occasionally, however, the take-it-easy comments made Claire distinctly uneasy. What if she didn't have such understanding parents, including a mother who had made it her mission to monitor Claire's moods and performance and to secure special accommodations precisely tailored to her every need? On one or two occasions when Claire teared up in class and sought refuge with the nurse or guidance counselor, she overheard the other kids complain that she needed to get herself together. Such comments angered her, but they nagged at her, too. From her parents' and doctors' explanations, she understood that she had a chemical imbalance in her brain that was just as real as any physical disability. Still, from time to time she wondered if she deserved all the breaks at school. It wasn't as if she was incapable of understanding the material or doing the work. Maybe, despite the reassuring people at the mental health conferences, she wasn't brave at all. Maybe, she thought, she was just lucky—a girl who had been given unusual privileges, who just couldn't hack it without all the extra scaffolding her parents, her doctor, and her school constructed for her.

On the other hand, Claire could justify the accommodations to herself based on one of the same qualities that likely made them palatable to the school: They were meant to fill in the gaps left by her medication. Her older brother and younger sister, both of whom responded quickly and dramatically to antidepressants, didn't require such measures. After all, Claire was "the real kid with depression."

CHAPTER 4

Early Rebellions

Drugs don't work in patients who don't take them.

—FORMER U.S. SURGEON GENERAL C. EVERETT KOOP,
AS QUOTED IN THE *New England Journal of Medicine,* 2005

In *Claire's Story,* the educational video about her experience with depression, thirteen-year-old Claire briefly discusses something that seems almost an aside: she doesn't like some of the side effects of medication, and once, thinking she was better, simply decided to stop taking it. But within days, she says in the voice-over, her depressive symptoms returned, and it became clear to her that she needed the drug after all. In fact, her suspicions returned from time to time. She'd get down on herself, concluding she was just whiny or bitchy and didn't need medication after all. As usual, her mother provided perspective, reminding Claire that her negative self-esteem and related doubts about her drug regimen were, in fact, a symptom of her depression. "Everyone feels that way sometimes about their medication, even your dad," Penny would say. The references to her schizophrenic father were enough to convince Claire. She had seen him in his relapses, and he was undeniably impaired. If even he could doubt the necessity of medication in the face of incontrovertible evidence, all because of his mental illness, then surely the same thing might be happening to her. Also, independent of these doubts, which she learned to attribute to a flare-up of her depression, Claire occasionally forgot to take her pill during her adolescence and continuing into her twenties—she sometimes even realized she had forgotten and didn't bother to go and fetch it, out of sheer laziness. But she never relinquished the drugs for any extended period of time, never resented her parents for pushing them on her. And in that way she was quite unusual, indeed.

Clinicians and researchers refer to the phenomenon of taking medication as prescribed as "compliance" or "adherence," with the latter thought to have somewhat less negative connotations. Such a definition leaves a lot of different ways to be nonadherent: failing to refill a prescription, quitting meds altogether, taking a higher or lower dose than prescribed, taking medication at different times than prescribed, taking one medication in a prescribed regimen but not another. The topic of adherence to medication of various kinds, not just psychotropic drugs, has attracted considerable attention from researchers and clinicians, the idea being that if you don't follow the doctor's orders, you are not maximizing your potential to get well. Despite this seemingly obvious proposition, a large percentage of patients, both young and old, do not adhere perfectly, even in the case of potentially life-saving interventions.

When Claire and her peers were first prescribed medication, in the 1990s, few studies existed examining young people's adherence to psychotropics. Those that did focused on adherence to stimulants and generally didn't distinguish between parents' decisions to take their children off medication and the children's own, private rebellions against their treatment. One notable exception, from 1982, found that 40 percent of ADHD children older than eight years old reported trying to avoid taking their meds, while fully 65 percent were known by parents or teachers to have tried to get out of taking the medications.[1] Parents' attitudes toward medication in younger children were probably more important in determining whether the children were actually taking the medication because of the simple fact that parents typically made the decisions about younger children's treatment. If they decided the treatment wasn't worth it, the child likely wasn't getting the pill—no matter how he or she personally felt about it.

Teenagers were another matter since, compared to younger kids, adults were likely to give them more responsibility over administering their own medications. Before the turn of the millennium, however, studies hadn't explicitly looked at adolescents' adherence. Since researchers knew that teenagers and adult psychiatric patients were the two groups with the lowest rates of compliance to medication regimens, they extrapolated that adolescent psychiatric patients would be especially unlikely to take their drugs as prescribed. Mental and emotional troubles at any age can cramp the mind's capacity to imagine consequences, including the ramifications of stopping one's medication. For young people who have yet to undergo the kind of cognitive development necessary for long-term planning, this handicap is coupled with the sense of the present as all consuming; everything in adolescence feels so immediate and important. It's hard to see why you ought to put up with current frustrations, like side effects, if you can't foresee long-term benefits. It's also easy to assume that if you feel a little better, you *are* better, or to reason, as the psychiatrist and psychotherapist Stephen Warres explained it to me, "I take medication, therefore I am sick. So if I do not take medication, then I would not be sick." Add this continuing short-term perspective to the normal adolescent urge to assert independence from adults, researchers theorized, and you would have a group of patients particularly prone to nonadherence.

Indeed, subsequent studies, the vast majority published after 2000, confirmed low, though widely variable, rates of adherence. Older kids were less likely than younger kids to take their drugs as prescribed. One study, for example, found that 72 percent of eleven-year-olds took medications more or less as prescribed, while only 32 percent of fifteen-year-olds did.[2] Presumably the higher rate of nonadherence among fifteen-year-olds is attributable to them being more responsible for overseeing their own treatment and more ready to rebel and assert their independence. Consistently, qualitative studies interviewing teenagers about their experiences of medication treatment showed the same thing: the older the child, the more likely they were to refuse the meds.

But to say that rebelling against one's medication is consistent with the normal trajectory of adolescent development isn't to minimize the motivations for it. The social work scholars Jeffrey Longhofer and Jerry Floersch have said that "adherence is always more than ingesting a pill"; similarly, nonadherence is always about more than *not* ingesting a pill.[3] The sociologist David Karp, who studies how people make sense of their psychotropic drugs, argues in his book *Is It Me or My Meds?* that teenagers have particularly good reason to question and doubt their medication, especially in a society like the United States, which sends young people infuriatingly mixed messages about how maturely they ought to behave and how much responsibility they are capable of assuming.[4] Feeling at once alienated from authority figures urging medication and powerless to direct the trajectory of their treatment, many teenagers assert their authority in one of the only ways they can: by refusing to take their medication in the manner their parents and doctors would like. Of course, they also chafe at medication for many of the same reasons adults do. Studies have shown that even quite young children, not to mention teenagers, worry about side effects.[5] Also, like adults, they don't always remember to take their pills, especially when meds such as stimulants and some older formulations of the atypical antipsychotics have to be taken multiple times a day. They may desire quick results that are not forthcoming; or they may simply become frustrated with trying one drug after another, without discernible change or improvement.

What may seem like a simple act of frustration or a developmentally normal assertion of independence, however, can also reflect a deeper, fundamental anxiety about what taking medications signifies, or about the ways in which it makes you "not yourself." At a time when the search for one's identity is already a fraught, challenging, and muddled process, rejecting drugs that change emotions and behavior can be not only a rebellion against authority figures, but an attempt to preserve the aspects of self kids hold dear. For Paul, the rebellion was stoked in his most restrictive placement yet, but the real impetus was how a particular drug challenged an image that he had worked hard to maintain.

Paul, ages ten to twelve
FORT LAUDERDALE, FLORIDA / 1998–2000

Before Paul landed in foster care, he had spent the first five years of his life in an environment where being cool and tough was the be-all and end-all, and he carried the street ethos with him into foster care. Even in homes in the fanciest neighborhoods, he lived life as though he were still in the ghetto, and impressed the sheltered suburban kids with his tough-guy pose. In a system where he had minimal control and no voice, image was everything. Ritalin and the mood-stabilizing anti-seizure drug Tegretol hadn't threatened that image because neither Paul nor his peers had perceived them having any effect on him. Seroquel, prescribed when Paul was ten for what his psychiatrists decided was bipolar disorder, produced side effects that constantly threatened the social persona he had painstakingly cultivated. This imperiled Paul's sense of himself.

For years, Paul went along taking medication because he didn't have a choice. The doctors prescribed increasing or decreasing doses for mysterious reasons, and his various foster parents doled them out, sometimes forgetting a dose, sometimes giving him too much by mistake or even on purpose, in what he interpreted as an effort to calm him down even more. He learned to use first Ritalin, and then Tegretol, as excuses for his bad behavior, attributing lapses or outbursts to a missed dose. But in truth he never noticed a difference in his mood or behavior with or without these two drugs. Seroquel, the antipsychotic drug doctors substituted for Tegretol after he overdosed in an attempt to convince his beloved foster parents to adopt him, was a different matter altogether.

Seroquel, newly on the market when Paul was prescribed it in the late 1990s, belonged to a new generation of psychiatric medications that drug companies had originally developed to treat schizophrenia. The older antipsychotics tamped down psychosis by heavily sedating the patient. They also caused troubling, sometimes permanent or long-lasting neurological side effects, including stiffness, trembling, and tics. These older antipsychotics, like Haldol and Thorazine, had developed a reputation as the blunt tools of mental institutions, and as those institutions emptied out in the 1970s and 1980s, the public saw the drugs' lasting effects up close, including the dull-eyed stare and stiff-limbed movements, the so-called "Thorazine shuffle." The terrible irony of these side effects was that the very drug that was supposed to make you well made you instantly recognizable as mentally ill.

The new drugs, dubbed atypical antipsychotics because they didn't produce the side effects of earlier antipsychotics, were hailed as revolutionary when they began appearing on the market in the late 1980s and early 1990s. The FDA first approved the drugs to treat the psychosis of schizophrenia, but doctors began prescribing them off-label to children and teenagers who were given the controversial new diagnosis of childhood bipolar disorder. Doctors and researchers had long thought that bipolar disorder didn't appear until at least the late teens, but in the 1980s some influential researchers began to argue that much of what was diagnosed as early-onset schizophrenia in children was in fact early-onset bipolar disorder. Symptoms of bipolar disorders manifested differently, they argued, in children and teenagers than they did in adults. In particular, young people were less likely to show the classic, well-demarcated cycles of mania and depression and were more likely to show erratic, rapidly shifting moods and behavior.

This new view quickly gained traction in the psychiatric establishment, and by 1997, the official treatment guidelines of the American Academy of Child and Adolescent Psychiatry noted: "Irritability, belligerence, and mixed manic-depressive features are more common than euphoria" and emphasized that the kinds of reckless behaviors typical of adult mania would be "limited to typical childhood behavior problems, such as school failure, fighting, dangerous play, and inappropriate sexualized activity." The problem, as these guidelines noted, was distinguishing these symptoms from those of other childhood disorders, like ADHD, oppositional defiant disorder, or conduct disorder, as well as from "the normal childhood phenomena of boasting, imaginary play, overactivity, and youthful indiscretions."[6]

The atypicals weren't prescribed only for bipolar disorder, however. Despite what many experts have criticized as meager evidence for wider use, doctors also began prescribing the drugs for aggression, agitation, impulsiveness, and self-injurious behavior, symptoms that could be associated with a range of behavior disorders. As a result, the rate of prescribing atypicals to children under twenty increased approximately sixfold between 1993 and 2002.[7] Yet, as was the case with antidepressants, prescriptions for atypicals accelerated without careful scientific studies judging their safety and efficacy in young people. The American Academy of Child and Adolescent Psychiatry's 1997 treatment guidelines noted that there were no studies demonstrating that antipsychotics were useful for treating bipolar children, and that it was in fact unclear whether they were effective at reducing mania, or whether they simply sedated young patients. As for the atypicals specifically, the guidelines cited a single case study of one teenager who had been reported to improve while taking them. The guidelines recommended lithium as a first-line treatment, and then the mood stabilizers Tegretol and Depakote.[8]

After Paul overdosed on Tegretol, however, his doctors apparently thought anticonvulsant drugs unwise and antipsychotics a better option, perhaps because the anticonvulsant mood stabilizers reach toxic levels more easily and therefore pose a greater risk of overdose. Seroquel, for reasons not explained to him, was the substitute. In fact, he took the medication for a couple of years before he was given a specific reason for its use. Paul had been complaining to his therapist at the behavioral school about how the medication made him feel—tired, dry-mouthed, sluggish—and how, at least when he first got to the school, his classmates teased him for taking a "crazy" drug after noticing his midday dosings (the teasing ended after Paul beat up enough kids). The therapist explained he'd been diagnosed a couple of years earlier with something called bipolar disorder, which meant that his moods and behaviors vacillated wildly and he needed something to balance them. Paul didn't find the explanation particularly salient. It seemed a variation of the same basic argument he'd been hearing since he went on Ritalin years before: that he was badly behaved and needed drugs to control him.

Studies published just a few years after Paul was prescribed Seroquel would show a strong link between childhood trauma and bipolar disorder that set in early and followed a more severe course.[9] Meanwhile, statistical analyses released both at the time he took medication and in the years afterward would show that foster-care children were medicated at a rate between three and eleven times that of their low-income peers on Medicaid, although white foster children were more likely to be medicated than minority children like Paul.[10] By the late 1990s reports were also appearing in the media questioning the circumstances under which foster children were receiving medication. The atypical antipsychotics, like Seroquel, were prescribed at an especially high rate.[11]

At age ten, Paul wasn't up in arms about his treatment on principle. In his world of group homes and behavior schools, medication was normal. He simply didn't like the way the Seroquel made him feel. He envisioned himself as tough, street-smart, devious, quick-witted. On the drug, he felt soft, groggy, slow. Sometimes the medication gave him double vision so that stationary objects appeared to be moving, and made him feel so out of it that on occasion he didn't even hear people talking to him. The science fiction film *The Matrix* came out in 1999, when Paul was eleven; the slow-motion scenes reminded him of how he felt when he took the Seroquel.

Seroquel, though it slowed him down, did not leave Paul feeling any more in control of his behavior; that is, he felt as in control as he had always felt. After being moved from Dan and Nora's, Paul was sent on a dizzying journey from one house to another. Sometimes, in a bid to be moved elsewhere, he deliberately vandalized the house or ran away, and sometimes the adults charged with his care maintained that they simply couldn't handle him. Either way, he was conscious of making a decision to act out, in hopes of getting out of each placement he disliked and eventually landing with a family who would love him unconditionally and adopt him.

Yet, with each transgression he moved through the foster-care system to stricter and stricter living arrangements with more intensive levels of psychiatric care. By middle school, he was living in group homes where almost all the children took a cocktail of strong medications. As he bounced from one placement to another, disingratiating himself not only with individual foster parents but with whole private companies with networks of homes, his case managers were running out of options. The last straw was his vandalization of a home in Miami. Paul's caseworker told him he was being transferred to a full-time care facility in Tampa, where there would be a working farm and staff specially trained to help him.

Paul had not counted on being moved to such a restrictive placement. He was now eleven and had been on Seroquel for a couple of years but was no longer taking Ritalin. Upon arriving in Tampa, he decided that he liked only two things about the facility: the girls and his classes, especially history, where they studied World War II. The girls seemed to like him too, but he thought the meds were hurting his game. Seroquel slowed him down, made him drool, and gave him red eyes. He didn't want to be like that with the girls he was trying to impress. For that, he had to be in cool-guy mode, not zombie mode. He started to wonder if he could find a way out of taking the drug.

So far as Paul could tell, every kid at the Tampa facility was on meds. It was, after all, a psychiatric treatment center. He liked his psychiatrist because, unlike previous doctors, he was good at listening and didn't try to put words in Paul's mouth. But clearly the facility was a big believer in medication. The nurses handed out the pills at breakfast, lunch, and again in the evening, and they watched to make sure Paul took them. Over time, though, Paul's good behavior won him some perks, including less stringent supervision when he took his pills. About three months into his stay, he started hiding the Seroquel under his tongue and then spitting it into a napkin that he'd later flush down the toilet. Occasionally, he judged it too risky not to swallow, but for the most part, he managed not to take his thrice-daily doses.

Without Seroquel, Paul felt like himself—energetic, social, the "alpha dog" at the Tampa facility. He worked out a lot and got a six-pack and a girlfriend. Even though he'd been told he had bipolar disorder and had no control over his moods or behavior, he was released from the facility after eight months. He'd been spitting out most doses of his meds for five months, but he wasn't surprised he'd managed to get out of the place without the help of medication. He'd never had much faith in it, and had always felt that ultimately, he was in charge of how he behaved. Now that he was back to group homes, it was anyone's guess if he'd be able to continue spitting out his pills, or if he'd have to go back to his overweight, sluggish self. It was all a question of the circumstances thrust upon him, and the ways he could find to dodge them.

In Paul's behavioral programs, medication was too ubiquitous to have much appeal. But in more typical school environments, certain meds have an allure, and kids and college students sold or gave away their drugs, especially stimulants and sedating antianxiety drugs, like Xanax. Doctors noticed, and many were on the alert when kids asked for too many refills or an unreasonably high dose. Diverting the drugs could be a rebellion, or just a giving-in; one young woman who was financially strapped in college described having to make the choice between saving her antianxiety meds for herself during exams, or selling them to freshmen who took them with alcohol to get a laid-back buzz. To a number of people I interviewed, learning that the drugs they'd been prescribed were so sought after for a high highlighted what they saw as the hypocrisy of their parents and doctors—and sometimes just how potent the drugs could be. "It brought pills to a whole different level in my consciousness, that they could be abused," one young woman from outside Boston said. "What did that mean? And how is it . . . different from just taking them orally with a prescription? And some people were just selling them to take them orally, so how is that different from just a doctor giving them to me?"

Abusing one's own medications can be a form of nonadherence, too, as can taking them with alcohol or other drugs. What little data exists, however, suggests that these activities are less common among younger adolescents than in people in their late teens and early twenties (children, interestingly, often dislike how they feel on too-high doses of stimulants). Overall, it's possible to think about young people's adherence to psychiatric medication as a cost-benefit analysis of whether the payoffs of taking medication are worth the sacrifices, in the form of side effects, hassle, stigma from peers, and so on. There is a fundamental conflict at the heart of med rebellions: the medications help kids gain a sense of control or agency over behaviors and emotions that they (or their adult minders) dislike, but to do so, they must submit to a drug, and, perhaps, even to being reliant upon it. Studies show that even when children identify as having a psychiatric disorder—and say they think their medication has helped improve their moods or behavior—they sometimes don't adhere to it because of side effects, peer stigma, or reluctance to rely on what they perceive as a chemical crutch.[12] But in Paul's mind there was no real cost-benefit analysis to be done, because he perceived no benefits from Seroquel. He didn't think he had a problem controlling his behavior, and he put little stock in the diagnosis of bipolar disorder. Rather, Seroquel symbolized to him all the myriad ways in which he felt disempowered in the foster-care and public mental-health systems.

The recurring lament of Paul's childhood was that no one ever listened to him or took his opinions seriously, and he felt the same was true with regard to his Seroquel treatment. It's worth noting that he was rarely without adults to confide in: he had therapists, sometimes one at school and one affiliated with his home placement, and also a so-called guardian *ad litem*, an adult volunteer who is supposed to represent the foster child's interests in court, and act as a mentor and ally. But Paul usually felt manipulated by his therapists, as though they were in cahoots with the prescribing doctors and trying to coerce him into saying what they wanted—that he had no control over his anger and aggression. His guardians *ad litem*, volunteers who were constantly in short supply, came and went. His favorite was an older man whom Paul initially wrote off (he considered the guy funny looking, with chicken legs and a huge belly). But Paul eventually grew close to him and confided his objections to the Seroquel. The guardian was sympathetic, but Paul also knew he was unlikely to lobby for a change in his psychiatric treatment. He had, after all, read Paul's case file, in which Paul was sure that all the adults reported that he was a terror, impossible to handle, not to mention that he had bipolar disorder. The forces in favor of medication seemed to him overwhelming.

Paul experienced much of his psychiatric care as oppressive and authoritarian, and in fact studies of teens' medication adherence confirm that kids who mistrust the people providing the medication are less likely to stick to their prescribed regimens. Other aspects of Paul's situation were typical of children who actively rebelled: many studies show that boys and ethnic minorities are less likely to take their meds, as are children with behavior disorders and boys who exhibit physical aggression.[13] The fact that Paul's rebellion occurred in the Tampa residential treatment center, his most restrictive placement yet, was probably not a coincidence, either. Tally Moses, who has studied teenagers' experiences of psychotropic medication in depth, argues that coercive medication treatment is particularly common in such settings, where staff struggle to maintain order and may aggressively medicate kids—especially with sedating antipsychotics like Seroquel—to suppress disturbing symptoms or aggressive behavior (Moses cites one study from 1998 in which more than half of eighty-three youths in a residential treatment center were given antipsychotics without solid diagnostic reasons).[14]

Paul's situation, both in the residential treatment center and in the foster-care system in general, was perhaps unusually oppressive compared to the experience of the average child on psychiatric medication. Yet, the power dynamic need not be so weighted as it was in Paul's case for children to be motivated to rebel. Small indignities and annoyances accumulate—round after round of doctor's appointments and prescriptions, daily monitoring and nagging parents, the lunchtime embarrassment of being fetched from class to take a pill. One young man who began taking ADHD medication as a third grader in Arizona and who cycled through a series of stimulants, antidepressants, and other drugs wrote to me, "If you named a time of day, there is a good chance [I] took meds during it . . . sometimes it was just in the morning, sometimes it was morning and lunch time, sometimes it was morning and evening . . . and rarely was it just one type of medication." His parents, he said, were always on him "like hawks" to take the pills, but whenever he got a chance—at sleepovers, playdates, religious youth group outings—he ditched the medications. (Summer camp was another matter: there the nurse carefully doled out the dosages to all the children taking meds.) His mini-rebellions were perhaps more transient acts of self-assertion, or a brief means of acting out after a series of accumulated frustrations, than any grand philosophical statement. That came later, in college, when he was in a better position to analyze the medications' effects on him and concluded they made him feel inhibited, tamped down his spontaneity and naturally goofy nature. But it was some time before he was willing to confess his decision to quit the medication to his parents. In ten years, they had never presented taking the drugs as a choice.

Other young people I interviewed, whose parents had allowed them to play a more active role in their treatment, recalled feeling less need to rebel. One young woman from Maryland named Mira, who was medicated with stimulants for attention problems in school when she was eight and then with antidepressants for depression a couple of years later, described a tense power dynamic with her parents over her obstinate behavior and poor grades, but a more flexible attitude toward her treatment. Indeed, her mother told me that the first day of Mira's Ritalin treatment, the pills gave her an awful headache and made her nauseous. Her mother was ready to give up then and there, but Mira insisted, saying she badly wanted to do better in school. Ritalin did improve her focus for a while, but then seemed to stop working. A second stimulant, Dexedrine, failed to work, and the antidepressant Paxil, prescribed in sixth grade for a lingering depression, caused alarming side effects, including obsessive picking at her skin that produced an open, infected wound on her scalp. Yet, with each proposed switch to a new medication, Mira's parents confirmed that she wanted to continue. Had they not done that, she suspects she would have rebelled, as one of her close friends did. But she badly wanted to get better, badly wanted to be happier and to please her parents by doing well in school, and that desire sustained her through one ineffective drug after another. Elizabeth, growing up in a nearby Maryland suburb, also wanted to do well in school, which may have helped sustain her commitment to Ritalin. But her relationship to antidepressants was another matter. Elizabeth was not sure she wanted to get better in the first place.

Elizabeth, ages fifteen to sixteen
MARYLAND SUBURBS OF WASHINGTON, DC / 1996–1997

From the time she was prescribed Ritalin and Prozac at the start of ninth grade, Elizabeth had taken what might be called a passive stance toward her medication. At first, her mother woke her up every morning and gave her both pills, but Liz usually couldn't find a convenient time to take her second Ritalin dose between classes, and often skipped or forgot it entirely. Then, partway through ninth grade, her mother stopped administering her morning dose, leaving it to Liz to remember, and checked in only rarely to see if she needed a refill. Some teenagers would have been happy with the autonomy. But Liz felt that both her parents—now occupied with the details of a separation agreement— were hands-off to the point of being oblivious. She felt abandoned and entrusted with more than she could handle. This was just one more instance where she was given too much responsibility, she thought—like the time in seventh grade when her parents announced on Christmas that they were splitting up and then left it up to Liz to decide whether the family should still spend New Year's together at their tiny timeshare in Florida. Now, without their supervision, she felt overwhelmed.

Perhaps even more important than the lack of supervision, though, was the lack of feedback about the medications' effects. It was, after all, the side effects of Ritalin, the nausea and wired feeling, that reminded her it had kicked in and made her notice that she was a bit more focused. Prozac's effects felt too amorphous. Had she discussed her treatment with her mother, or in more depth with her doctor, she might have realized that she was likely taking too low a dose of Ritalin for it to help her significantly, and been able to tell that either her moods had improved on Prozac or they hadn't, in which case it might be worth trying a different antidepressant, since only about a third of patients respond positively to the first antidepressant they try. But Liz's mother was distracted and stressed out, her father largely checked out (not to mention responsible, in Liz's opinion, for breaking up the family), and her relationship with her psychiatrist was limited at best.

Indeed, although she told her mother during the fall of tenth grade that she no longer wanted to take Prozac, she blanched at the prospect of confessing to her psychiatrist. The regular fifteen-minute med-check appointments were agonizing enough. Though she had made more friends during ninth and tenth grade, becoming more socially adroit, once she entered a therapist or psychiatrist's office she'd just stare at the books and knickknacks and clam up completely. She felt like she couldn't force words out of her mouth even if she'd wanted to. Now, embarrassed at having failed to follow the psychiatrist's prescription and unable to explain why, even to herself, she wanted to open up even less. If this was a rebellion against anything—against her medication, against psychiatry, against her parents, against who-knows-what—it wasn't a rebellion she wanted to acknowledge, let alone be forced to discuss and defend. The prospect of telling the psychiatrist was so daunting, in fact, that she threatened her mother with ditching the Ritalin, too, unless her mom found her a new doctor. As usual, her mother capitulated. When Liz saw the new doctor, she casually mentioned she'd previously taken Prozac, but that she was fine without it.

Liz wasn't necessarily rejecting antidepressants for good when she let them run out during the fall of tenth grade, but as time went on she simply didn't seek a refill, even as she began to sink into a deep depression. Around the same time, she befriended a circle of classmates who, even more than her pals at camp, thrived on interpersonal drama and embraced their identity as "fucked-up kids." Several of them had taken to cutting themselves in secret, which, as Liz gleaned, helped put their emotional pain into something tangible. In theory, she found the practice disturbing, but a few months after she went off Prozac, she took to cutting herself occasionally, too. It turned out to be an effective way of calming herself.

So-called "cutting," otherwise variously referred to as self-injury, self-harm, and self-mutilation, was by no means a new phenomenon in the 1990s, although it was undergoing increasing scrutiny: Johnny Depp and Princess Diana had both admitted to self-injury, a psychotherapist published a young adult novel about the subject called *The Luckiest Girl in the World*, and the *New York Times Magazine* ran a lengthy article on the topic in 1997. The article profiled a girl who had begun cutting herself, been treated with Prozac for depression and improved, but had gone off the medication after a few months and resumed the practice.[15]

Liz didn't cut frequently, just when the tension built up to a point she couldn't bear. She was careful to cut only when it was cold enough to wear long-sleeved shirts to cover the wounds. But her despair during this time, in tenth and eleventh grade, wasn't unrelenting. At times when she felt more cheerful, she couldn't remember quite how it felt to be depressed, but nevertheless felt a twinge, as though her past unhappiness were calling her back. "I realized I still want to be depressed," she wrote in a diary entry from her junior year. "Like if you are, it proves you're a real person, and if I'm always happy, it means I don't really feel things. Anyway, I guess I romanticize depression. Which is funny, because I don't enjoy it when I am. More like I like the idea of it."

She had good company. Much scholarship, far more than can be examined here, illuminates how Western culture in particular has romanticized and fetishized depression. Plato regarded poetry as a form of divine madness; one of Shakespeare's more famous speeches proclaims, "The lunatic, the lover, and the poet / Are of imagination all compact." The privileged perspective of melancholy became even more pronounced in the age of Romantic *Sturm und Drang*, Keats's "Ode on Melancholy," and Puccini's sad outcasts. The psychiatrist Peter Kramer, who traces this tradition of "heroic melancholy" back two thousand years in his book *Against Depression*, argues that the mythologizing of melancholy is largely an attempt to make sense of it in the face of nonexistent or ineffectual treatments. Perhaps so, but this doesn't account for its celebration from fifteenth-century Italy to sixteenth-century Elizabethan England to the Romantics of the nineteenth century to music genres such as grunge and emo at the end of the twentieth. The attraction to the melancholic persists, Kramer writes, even with the end of "therapeutic impotence," notably the flood of alleged wonder drugs, because it represents rebellion against "the seductions of bourgeois satisfactions."[16] Even Liz and her peers, growing up in an age of unabashed psychopharmacological and economic exuberance, a time the federal government called "the Decade of the Brain," felt this allure. Grunge, and youth culture in general, prominent through the first half of the decade, also fetishized the alienated, apathetic slacker and undoubtedly held a lot more sway over kids than the headlines or evening news segments about wonder drugs and brain-scanning findings.

One need not thoroughly romanticize misery, though, to become attached to it. Elizabeth Wurtzel, in her 1994 book *Prozac Nation*, is stridently critical of the urge to airbrush depression, yet she writes, "In a strange way, I had fallen in love with my depression. . . . I loved it because I thought it was all I had. I thought depression was the part of my character that made me worthwhile. I thought so little of myself, felt that I had such scant offerings to give to the world, that the one thing that justified my existence at all was my agony."[17] But ultimately, her book, in its rapturous self-absorption and with the picture of its pretty, pouting author on the cover, does serve to glamorize depression.

This lingering flirtation with the authenticity and depth that depression seems to produce, and the suspicion that the medications might erase it, is not, of course, particular to teenagers. Yet, having gone through it myself at the same age, I would argue that depression holds particular appeal for adolescents (upon reading *Hamlet*, I was disappointed to learn from my English professor parents that the character, despite his tortured search for self, seemingly so evocative of adolescence, is in fact thirty years old). Now, I can look back and dismiss my own infatuation with melancholy as a phase, but I am also acutely aware that the choice to move beyond, to embrace medication, was mine to make. Liz, however, was led to treatment at a time when she was still drawn to the seductive idea of being a tortured, "fucked-up" teenager with unfathomable depths of sorrow. Even after she had given up her drama-prone group of friends and stopped cutting herself, she kept being called back to the allure of misery. During the fall of her senior year, she wrote a poem that she tucked away in a school notebook:

> *Madness floats by in a cloud*
> *and I rush to catch it*
> *longing to be surrounded in mist*
> *as the wind splits the sky*
> *so I blow bubbles*
> *and pretend I'm insane.*
> *Because I used to be*
> *and I miss it.*

Despite her ongoing attraction to the melancholic, Liz found the reality of depression unpleasant enough that she had begun to consider going back on antidepressants during her junior year, after the school told her parents she had been cutting herself. Though she felt less morbid, she was overwhelmed with anxiety, something she thought of as a symptom of her depression, as opposed to a condition in its own right. Stressed out about academics, looming SATs, and the next year's college applications, she had a panic attack outside her school's main building as her mother was coming to pick her up. Alarmed, her mother insisted that Liz see her psychiatrist at once. But Liz had been telling this psychiatrist that she wasn't depressed. Now that it was time to confess, she felt like the little girl who cried wolf. She told him she'd had a panic attack. "It wasn't a panic attack. You're fine," the doctor said, and prescribed some more Ritalin. She could, of course, have gone straight to another doctor and come clean about everything and likely landed a refill of her Prozac. But having been shot down once, she delayed for months. She discussed the prospect at length with her boyfriend, and with his encouragement finally got up the courage to go to a new psychiatrist, confess her history, and ask for a prescription.

As different as Paul's and Liz's cases and upbringings are, they have several common traits: rejection of medication, hostility to psychiatric care in general, and lack of a close, long-term relationship with a doctor they trusted. Liz's mother let her call the shots with regards to whether she continued to see a given doctor, but rather than feeling empowered, Liz felt as if she had been set adrift, without anyone providing her outside feedback on how she was faring on medication, or, crucially, giving her a chance to discuss her hesitations and misgivings about continuing treatment. Liz disliked "shrinks," as she called talk therapists, and had a horror of explaining to her prescribing psychiatrist why she had quit Prozac. But it's possible that if she had seen the psychiatrist for more than fifteen-minute "med checks" every few months, she would have been more comfortable disclosing how she felt about her medication, elaborating the ways in which she both had trouble gauging its effects and also tended to romanticize her depression when she was feeling better. And even if she hadn't confessed these misgivings, at least she would have been seeing someone regularly who was aware of her depression and watching for signs that she was relapsing or cutting herself.

Her lack of faith in doctors hurt her, too, when she decided she did want medication treatment, after all. The doctor didn't know her well, and discredited her reports of depression and panic attacks and her belief that she needed something besides Ritalin. As was the case for Paul, not being taken seriously further undermined Liz's trust in the mental health profession, delaying her from seeking out a new psychiatrist willing to prescribe an antidepressant. Ostensibly, unlike Paul, she was in control of her treatment—she was responsible for taking her own pills, for letting her mother know when she had run out, and for choosing when and whether she saw a psychiatrist or therapist. Yet in effect, like Paul, she was left to fend for herself, with little guidance.

And, during a time when treatment was shifting toward brief med checks, or of bifurcated care involving med checks by an MD and talk therapy or cognitive-behavioral therapy by a psychologist, social worker, or other counselor, Liz's situation was hardly unique. So long as treatment is going well, and a young person is committed to it, long discussions about attitudes toward medication may not be necessary. But given that young people, especially if they feel treatment is forced upon them, are likely to rebel against their medications, more careful monitoring than what Liz received is often justified. I interviewed one child and adolescent psychiatrist in Maryland who makes her patients sign a pledge at the beginning of treatment promising they will not quit their medications without at least alerting her and explaining why. She tells kids that she won't immediately write them off if they decide they want to abandon their medications—she values their opinion—but that quitting randomly is simply too dangerous to do on their own.

I did interview a number of young people, however, who did not have close relationships with their prescribers but who nevertheless did not quit their medication on their own. A cursory relationship with a doctor does not guarantee a cursory relationship with medication (indeed, in college I was the one pushing to continue medication treatment, while my pediatrician, whom I only saw perhaps a couple of times a year, was urging a break). But combined with other factors—an absence of communication with parents, a sense of not having control over their circumstances—the lack of a close patient-doctor relationship can increase the likelihood that kids will give up their medication, and that when they do, potentially dangerous outcomes, like Elizabeth's cutting, will go unnoticed.[18]

As is the case for strong therapeutic relationships, studies show that positive, supportive family ties also increase the likelihood of kids' adhering to their treatment. Young people who have a greater sense of autonomy and more trust in adults' treatment decisions are less likely to perceive treatment as coerced.[19] Conversely, less family support, greater family conflict, and parents who are indifferent, over- or underinvolved, or struggling with their own psychological problems correlate with poor adherence.[20]

One might think that kids who start medication in childhood would by adolescence have resigned themselves to the long-term nature of the treatment and would need less external reinforcement. Some studies, indeed, have found that children who begin treatment at a younger age are more likely to continue taking their medication, though it's also likely that parental commitment to the drugs plays a role. Children who started medication earlier may have had parents who were more enthusiastic about treatment and perhaps more generally watchful and involved in their children's care, while those who began taking them later may have had parents who were ambivalent about treatment. Some recent, as-yet-unpublished findings from social science surveys of college students indicate, for example, that those with a father who openly disapproved of medication were less likely to adhere to it.[21]

It's true that for many kids, including a number I interviewed, adherence becomes routine over time; they take the pills almost unthinkingly, as they might vitamins. Some qualitative research on kids' experience of medication bears this out. "I don't really feel the medicine anymore," a fourteen-year-old girl told researcher Tally Moses in her study of teenagers' commitment to continuing their medications. "I'm sure it's helping me in some way. . . . Like I started taking medication for ADHD when I was five years old so it's not like it's new. I've pretty much lived with it for as long as I can remember."[22] Nevertheless, for many kids at this age, the drugs contribute to a sense of constantly grasping and questing after one's identity, of being involved in a very immediate and intense process of self-discovery that leads to more introspection and questioning, even in the case of long-lasting treatment. In addition to asking what purpose the medication is serving and how well it is achieving that purpose, teenagers can quite legitimately ask another question: "Am I still the same person who needed medication back then?"

Alex, ages ten to eighteen
LONG ISLAND AND BROOKLYN, NEW YORK / 1998–2006

By the end of high school, Alex would have said he was definitely not the same person who needed medication back in elementary and middle school. He wasn't even sure he had needed it then, in fact. Looking back, it seemed to him that he'd been just another coddled, "overmedicated kid" when he had taken an antidepressant to treat obsessive thoughts and behaviors between the ages of ten and fifteen. He had tapered off with his mother's and doctor's approval and therefore hadn't rebelled against meds in the way many other children did. As he looked back on his treatment from age eighteen, he began to think it had been unnecessary.

Alex had never questioned the meds while he was taking them, in part because he was a naturally obliging and mild-mannered child, and in part because his troubles had come on so suddenly that for years he considered them almost like an infection that required medication to be eradicated. The thoughts had appeared seemingly out of the blue one morning in 1998, the day after Alex's mother, a registered nurse, and her boyfriend, who had been living with the family for the past several months, got back from a birthday trip to Acapulco. Glad to have his mother back, Alex was all ready to leave for the Catholic parish school he attended when the thoughts invaded his head: *What if*, he wondered, *I'm not my mom's son after all? What if I'm adopted?*

Alarmed, he told his mother immediately. Despite her reassurances, the question stayed lodged in his brain. After a week or so, she took him to a psychiatrist. On hearing about Alex's recent worries and his history of compulsive straightening, checking, and neatening, the psychiatrist diagnosed obsessive-compulsive disorder (OCD) and recommended treatment with medication. Though Alex didn't know it at the time, the doctor also diagnosed generalized anxiety disorder and depression.

OCD wasn't one of the more common anxiety disorders in either adults or children. It was believed to occur in about 1 percent of the population, compared to perhaps 6 percent of kids thought to suffer from separation anxiety disorder, an intense upset at being apart from one's parents. But OCD was getting increased attention in the 1990s thanks to some surprisingly effective new treatments and a 1989 best-seller, *The Boy Who Couldn't Stop Washing*, by Judith Rapoport, who headed the National Institute of Mental Health's child psychiatry branch. As Rapoport's book explained, prior to the late 1980s OCD had been one of the most frustrating disorders for doctors and researchers: there was no effective treatment, either for children or adults. The most promising pharmaceutical option, a tricyclic antidepressant called Anafranil, was available in the United States only to researchers who received special permission from the government. By 1998, when Alex was diagnosed, Anafranil had been approved for seven years, and the new SSRI antidepressants were also showing promise for treating OCD.

Luvox, the drug that Alex was prescribed, was one of the so-called "me-too" SSRIs that came on the market in the early 1990s as pharmaceutical companies raced to develop their own versions of Prozac, Eli Lilly's blockbuster, multipurpose antidepressant. In 1997, Luvox became the first SSRI approved for treating OCD in children and teenagers.[23] Studies of OCD during the 1990s had also empirically demonstrated the effectiveness of cognitive-behavioral therapy, or CBT, a short-term form of therapy that focuses on revising and diffusing thoughts and behaviors believed to contribute to psychiatric symptoms. Alex received two years of therapy that seems to have incorporated elements of CBT, but he didn't feel close to his therapist and didn't see a connection between her suggestions and his feeling any better.

Alex's obsessive thoughts didn't go away immediately, and it took the psychiatrist perhaps a year to get him to a therapeutic dose of Luvox. But the obsessions gradually dominated his thinking less, and his compulsions also began to recede, so that he eventually allowed himself to read each sentence in a book just three times in a row, for example, instead of ten. He was doing so much better, in fact, that when his aunt and three cousins moved into the family's small house after a real estate deal went bad, Alex didn't even mind sharing a room with his cousin, a real slob.

Even more strikingly, when his father died of complications relating to obesity the next December, Alex weathered the loss well enough to wonder why he wasn't feeling more upset. Years later, with the benefit of therapy, he reasoned that his muted reaction wasn't so strange after all since he had never felt close to his father, who was already married with a child when Alex was born. During his weekly visits, his father would sit awkwardly in the living room of Alex's mom's house while they watched TV. It seemed to Alex that there was never anything to talk about.

Alex had always been a loner, and the medication didn't change that, although at the time SSRIs were gaining a lot of attention for their ability to treat a relatively new and controversial condition, social anxiety disorder. Neither Luvox nor his two years in CBT changed Alex's personality or enabled him to develop skills for making friends at his parish school or the elite all-boys' Catholic school that he began attending in ninth grade. His continuing social seclusion didn't bother him much, though; he was proud of his excellent academic record, and thought it would have been far worse to embarrass himself by reaching out to his peers and being rejected. In ninth grade, some of the tension at home eased when his mother's boyfriend, with whom Alex had clashed whenever Alex's lingering need for order compelled him to straighten up around the house, moved out. In tenth grade, Alex seemed sufficiently calm and well adjusted that he, his mom, and the psychiatrist all agreed that he should see how he fared without the medication.

Such decisions were common practice among doctors eager to avoid indefinite pharmaceutical treatment for young people. "*No child should remain on medication for more than a year without his doctor considering a medication-free period* to assess whether or not he still needs such treatment," the prominent child psychiatrist David Fassler advised parents in a 1997 book.[24] Although in its most severe forms OCD could be a lifelong, debilitating illness, many childhood anxiety disorders were known to wax and wane. In its 1998 treatment guidelines, the American Academy of Child and Adolescent Psychiatry recommended continuing treatment for twelve to eighteen months after the child's acute symptoms were resolved and then testing how the child fared without medication, though the authors emphasized that studies showed most children and adults relapsed within a few months.[25]

About a year after Alex had stopped taking Luvox, his mother was getting serious with a new boyfriend, Tony. Within a few months they were engaged, and by the summer they were married. Alex's checking and cleaning habits had never totally abated even when he was taking medication. Where his mother's former boyfriend had simply complained when Alex moved his stuff, Tony liked to provoke Alex by deliberately messing things up around the house after Alex had tidied up. They went back and forth in a constant, maddening cycle: Alex would straighten a pile of books, Tony would mess it up. Alex would complain to his mom, and soon they'd all be yelling at each other. The relationship grew more and more strained, with Tony complaining that Alex was a mama's boy who needed to earn money to support himself, and Alex feeling that Tony didn't appreciate his academic accomplishments.

Overall, Alex thought Tony a brute and a bully who was emotionally abusive toward both Alex and his mother, whom Tony worked to isolate from her parents and siblings. Nonetheless, Alex began to consider one of Tony's common gripes justified: American society was too quick to medicate—especially in the case of children's psychological and behavioral problems. An epileptic who refused to take his medication in order to feel self-sufficient, Tony believed in mental and physical toughness. Tony knew Alex had taken an antidepressant, and though Alex didn't take Tony's comments as jibes at him in particular, he did think that he might have been capable of avoiding Luvox. Even if he had needed the medication back then, he told himself, he didn't need it any longer. He was different now: tougher, more seasoned, more independent.

Alex considered Tony easily the worst thing in his life, but was proud that for the past several years he had survived the emotional abuse sans medication. As senior year wore on and Alex prepared to attend a nearby private college, which he'd pay for himself with loans and money earned from part-time jobs, Tony seemed to ease up on his bullying. As Alex saw it, there was no reason to think he would need medication again. Within a few months, he would know how wrong he had been.

CHAPTER 5

Something New?

Throughout most of her adolescence, the signs had been there:
I simply hadn't seen them.

—COLETTE DOWLING,
New York Magazine, JANUARY 20, 1992

As she pored over childhood photographs of her daughter, the writer
Colette Dowling was haunted. Years after the photos were taken, when
her daughter was in her early twenties, the young woman suffered an
acute episode of depression. The photos "revealed a somberness, a melancholy, as if the camera had caught something too fleeting for us to
see in a girl—a talented student and athlete, who was clearly on the fast
track," Dowling wrote. "If she'd been evaluated earlier, her psychiatrist
says, she could have been spared several episodes of illness."

The year was 1992, and the article in *New York Magazine* was titled
"Rescuing Your Child from Depression."[1] It was full of the enthusiasm
that characterized much of the era's writing about the new generation of
SSRI antidepressants. Unlike Dowling's daughter, who had been born
too early to benefit from the latest advances in child psychopharmacology, children of the 1990s did not need to endure years of suffering from
mood and anxiety disorders.

Moreover, mounting evidence demonstrated that untreated mental
illness, especially illness that began in childhood or adolescence, posed

serious long-term risks. Derived from observations that depression was a recurring illness that tended to worsen over time, the "kindling" hypothesis held that each subsequent episode put the sufferer at risk of more, and more severe, episodes down the road. Clinicians also noted that although an initial episode of depression was often linked to some external stressor, successive episodes occurred with seemingly milder and milder triggers, so that depression, with time, seemed to take on a life of its own. At the National Institute of Mental Health, researchers Robert Post and Susan Weiss hypothesized that, as is the case in many seizure disorders, each episode changes the wiring of the brain, sensitizing it to smaller and smaller stressors. A similar phenomenon might hold true for mania and perhaps anxiety disorders, they speculated.[2] On the basis of this theory, early intervention for depression and perhaps other conditions seemed wise, and lifelong treatment might be warranted if one or more trial periods without drugs resulted in a relapse.

Yet treatment was not often so simple as nipping a disorder in the bud, or implementing a no-meds trial to test for relapse. Even if young people were correctly diagnosed—and that is a big if, given the vagaries of diagnosis and the difficulty of distinguishing normal development from pathology—medications could stop working, and symptoms could change over time as the child matured. A child diagnosed and medicated for an anxiety disorder might indeed grow out of it, as some disorders disappear altogether by adolescence or adulthood. Or the patient might appear improved, only to develop new symptoms. Were these symptoms a recurrence of the original disorder, or something else altogether? In some cases it didn't much matter, since anxiety and depression, for example, are both treated with antidepressants. But in other cases, new symptoms presented a therapeutic dilemma. A child with ADHD would typically be treated with stimulants, but a child with bipolar disorder with mood stabilizers or antipsychotics. Stimulants, though, can exacerbate or even precipitate mania, and each successive manic episode seemed to put a person at risk of others. Hence, a misdiagnosis could have serious implications for a young person's long-term prognosis.

The phenomena of evolving illness and breakdowns (discussed, respectively, in this chapter and the next) can be extremely discouraging to a high-functioning person who has been taking meds for much of her youth. Fighting mental illness often turns out to be an ongoing battle with new symptoms and new drugs, a constant adjustment that kids, as well as their parents, could have never foreseen when they began taking medication. While many found their situation less dire than it had been without drugs, many also discovered, to their dismay, that the new psychotropic medications do not eradicate, and indeed can sometimes exacerbate, mental illness. Since the most widely prescribed psychiatric drugs had not yet been tested in young people by years of accumulated clinical experience or far-reaching, longitudinal medical studies, prescribing doctors and their patients simply did not know enough about how these drugs work, or what their long-term effects would be, to predict how they would work years, or sometimes weeks or even days, in the future.

Changing diagnoses and modes of treatment have serious implications for a child's self-discovery or a teenager's identity development. For some young people, the label and the prescription change so frequently that they are constantly unsure of the nature of their problems and their abilities. Others, myself included, have felt confident that they had everything figured out, only to experience symptoms that felt shockingly different, sometimes finding that medication no longer did them any good. That's what happened to Caleb when, four years after Zoloft rescued him from a severe depression, he began to feel strangely exhilarated.

Caleb, ages twelve to eighteen
TRI-CITIES, WASHINGTON / 1996–2002

Caleb was born and raised in eastern Washington State, near where both his parents had spent their childhoods. His grandparents had come to the region when it was booming during World War II, and his parents both worked at the large government laboratory that dominated the region's employment sector: his father a scientist working on national security technologies, and his mother in communications. His parents were cautious regarding medical treatment, wary of what was not scientifically proven.

When Caleb, their only child, was about nine, he began having seizures. They didn't last long—about a minute, but he'd stumble around and drool and would emerge from them having no idea how long he'd been out. Not long before, his maternal grandfather had died of a brain tumor, and his parents, now on high alert for neurological symptoms, brought Caleb to a local neurologist who prescribed an anticonvulsant medication. Anticonvulsants, which reduce electrical activity in the brain, are also commonly used as mood stabilizers for bipolar disorder.

Caleb's father, who had suffered seizures briefly as a child but outgrew them, was generally wary of confining his son to a "drug-induced haze," while his mother worried about the possible long-term effects (gum malformations are one for the drug Caleb ended up taking). Following the neurologist's advice, his parents put him on the anticonvulsant temporarily, but took him to a pediatric neurologist in Seattle for a second opinion. The neurologist, who saw thousands of children a year, said the drug probably wasn't necessary since, like his dad, Caleb would probably outgrow the seizures. Caleb's parents gratefully took him off the drug, and sure enough, the seizures went away on their own.

Four years later, his parents reacted quite differently to the prospect of medication. One day, as the family was dining at a bright and cheerful taqueria, Caleb broke down crying. He couldn't bear it anymore, he said. He desperately needed help for the depression that had overtaken him. His symptoms had begun about a year earlier, shortly after he transferred to an all-boys' Christian school at the beginning of seventh grade. Though he had gotten along well with children at his old school, his new classmates, many of whom had gone to school together for years, treated him as an interloper. Caleb was still small, not having hit his growth spurt, and was bullied mercilessly and frequently beaten up. Far worse than the actual beatings, however, was the anticipation of them reoccurring. The other boys threatened to kill him so often that after a time Caleb came to believe them. Partway through eighth grade, he begged his parents to let him transfer back to public school, and although they agreed, it seemed already too late to lift him out of his all-consuming depression.

At the private school Caleb had felt alternately panicky, overwhelmed, and hopeless about the world holding anything for him but his current, painful gloom. Now, as if to protect himself, he had stopped feeling anything at all. He slept about sixteen hours a day, more if he could, and awoke feeling as though he'd scarcely dozed. He did as little as possible, and neglected his health and hygiene—even shaving his head so that he wouldn't have to wash his hair. Affectless and apathetic, he spoke without inflection, in monosyllables. And he became fearless. Once terrified by threats to kill him, he now felt, like Keats, "half in love with easeful death." Fantasizing about killing himself gave him an out from the exhausting, oppressive weight of living.

His parents, who worked long hours at the laboratory, had known he was being bullied at his old school. But, like many parents whose children had internalizing disorders like depression and anxiety, as opposed to behavior disorders, they had underestimated their son's devastation, at least until that night at the taqueria when he told them outright that he couldn't go on. As his desperation spilled out amid the bustling crowd happily enjoying their tacos and enchiladas, they could tell he needed help—immediately. They took him to both a psychologist and a psychiatrist, both of whom said Caleb's was one of the worst cases of major depressive disorder they had ever seen. The psychiatrist prescribed Zoloft, an SSRI antidepressant that had come on the market a few years earlier.

This time around, in contrast to the episode four years before with the antiseizure medication, Caleb's parents didn't question the prescription. The way he had articulated his symptoms so perfectly—virtually diagnosed himself—indicated the urgency of his need for an intervention. Since Caleb had also been diagnosed with post-traumatic stress disorder due to the severe bullying he had endured at his old school, they also arranged for weekly cognitive-behavioral therapy with a psychologist.

Caleb credited the therapy with helping to contain the anxiety and stave off the flashbacks of bullying that overcame him in crowded places, but he considered the Zoloft truly transformative. Just a couple of weeks after beginning treatment, Caleb was sitting in his psychiatrist's waiting room when suddenly he noticed a white-noise machine purring at him. Had it been there all along, he wondered? Had the psychiatrist put it there to calm people down before their appointments? Then he caught himself, realizing that for the first time in months, he was able to concentrate on something besides his own despair. One night, when he woke up and got out of bed to go to the bathroom, he was overwhelmed by the soft texture of the carpet against his feet, brought to tears by the sense that he could finally experience the world again.

During the next few weeks, Caleb actually began to look forward to some things—food, nice smells, or a good joke. Colors looked brighter. In school, he could not only concentrate again but found himself actually interested in the subject matter. His peers no longer kept a cautious distance as they had when he was at his lowest. He began to make friends.

Caleb remained on Zoloft through high school. He never expected to cease medication because he never expected to escape his depression. Even after his remarkable turnaround in eighth grade, he retained a gloomy fatalism: the medication might keep him afloat for now, but he was always in danger of drowning. Every few months, he was very nearly submerged by his depression, which swept him up like a giant wave, immersing him in pockets of familiar and hopeless misery. He'd hear a voice, always speaking the same commanding imperative: *End it now*, it would say. *Do it now!* Caleb succeeded in batting away the thoughts, and after a few days, the misery would lift. Yet it always returned to remind him that Zoloft was perhaps the only thing standing between him and oblivion. He assumed he would be on medication for the rest of his life.

Then, during his senior year, his mood shifted. For the past four years, he had been content simply to enjoy the ordinary pleasures of being a teenager, like learning to drive. But as his senior year progressed, he grew restless. Having lost so much time to his depression, and having thought for years that he wouldn't make it out of high school alive, he now felt an increasing sense of urgency. *Why the hell am I still alive?* he'd ask himself. *I must be here for a reason. I gotta start accomplishing shit. Now that I've gone through all this pain, what can I take from it and make good? How can I grow a rose from concrete?*

While his classmates indulged their senioritis, Caleb, still taking

Zoloft, proceeded at a breakneck pace. He couldn't say for sure what he was racing toward, though he had some idea of going into engineering or another scientific field where he might build grand structures or make momentous discoveries. He attended a trade school in the mornings to study computer programming and regular high school classes in the afternoons. At daily track practice, he ran himself ragged training for the four-hundred-meter race, an event requiring grueling endurance, explosive strength, and high speed. In the evenings, he attended classes at the local community college. He slept and ate very little, but found himself neither tired nor hungry. He noticed, too, that he was beginning to speak quickly, and that when he laughed the sheer force of his guffawing seemed to overpower him, as if excess electricity were coursing through his body. His skin felt prickly, and he didn't want to be touched. His parents took to teasing him about his solitary, macho-man posture by singing the Simon and Garfunkel song "I Am a Rock."

Caleb brushed them off, but didn't deny the accuracy of the message. He did feel invincible. This wasn't merely a lifting of his depression, he realized by the end of his senior year. It was something else altogether, though what he wasn't sure. He wondered, as he had when his depression set in six years earlier, whether he was merely going through some new phase of puberty, some hormonal shift that was throwing his emotions and his body out of whack. He even asked his father about it one day. His dad looked at Caleb, young, tan, muscled, with a driven look in his eyes, and seemed at a loss about what to say. He seemed better than healthy; what could be wrong?

After graduation, Caleb enrolled full-time at the local community college and continued to live at home with his parents at their cozy split-level house in a development on the north side of town. On a visit to his psychiatrist that summer, Caleb announced that, contrary to his expectations, his depression seemed to have vanished altogether, and he wanted to try going off Zoloft. His psychiatrist raised his bushy eyebrows and peered at Caleb skeptically over his glasses. Reluctantly, he agreed, but insisted that Caleb continue to see him for monitoring. Caleb, feeling more restless than ever, was glad to be moving on. Later, he'd understand the real reasons for his newly inflated mood. For the time being, he was elated to be free of the medication he'd thought he'd need for the rest of his life.

As an adult, Caleb couldn't remember whether his psychiatrist had presented Zoloft, or antidepressants in general, as an indefinite commitment back when he first wrote the prescription in 1998. At that time, triage for child and adolescent depression recommended prescribing medication for nine months or a year and then seeing how the child fared without it, to avoid the prospect of unnecessary long-term treatment (in fact, the first randomized controlled study of multiyear antidepressant treatment for adolescents with major depression didn't come out until 2008).³ But Caleb suffered so many relapses, even on medication, that his doctor never suggested a medication-free trial. Since each relapse increased the likelihood that Caleb was facing an intractable, and probably lifelong, illness, Caleb's psychiatrist was deeply skeptical when, four years after beginning the medications, Caleb suddenly announced that he felt cured. In fact, the doctor had good reason to suspect that this radical transformation, having occurred while Caleb was taking an antidepressant, might suggest he was suffering from another disorder altogether.

In the fall of 2002, having been free of Zoloft for several months, Caleb was taking his second term of community college classes when he began to feel hyper, his default setting a few notches too high. Sometimes it was great—he'd go for drives at high speeds, listening to songs with pounding, relentless beats. At times, he felt sickeningly restless, as if he wanted to jump out of his skin. He experienced unnerving out-of-body sensations, as though he were a movie director instructing his body how to act. He'd take in data from everywhere, without even wanting to, noticing the numbers on stock tickers or information on flyers and billboards. Toward the end of the semester, Caleb tried to tell his psychiatrist what was happening, but found himself unable to articulate exactly what felt so wrong. Still, the doctor agreed that the no-medication experiment hadn't worked out well and prescribed a different kind of antidepressant, called Effexor, which had come out a couple of years after Zoloft and which worked on two neurotransmitter systems in the brain—both serotonin and norepinephrine—instead of serotonin alone. The doctor may have prescribed it because he feared that Caleb's high-wire sensations were more likely to be exacerbated by Zoloft and other SSRIs. When Effexor too sent Caleb spinning into mania, the doctor finally sat him down for a reassessment. "I think," he said, "that you may have had a few manic episodes."

When Caleb's psychiatrist made this suggestion, around 2003, clinicians had long known that both adults and children often suffered from psychiatric comorbidity, the presence of more than one psychological disorder. But they also knew that symptoms of a given disease could change over a lifespan, and that comorbid conditions do not necessarily arrive simultaneously. That left the question of whether a child diagnosed with first one condition and then another had two different disorders, or whether the first might be a misdiagnosed early form, or "prodrome," of the second. In the 1990s, for example, researchers noticed a high rate of overlap between ADHD and childhood bipolar disorder, with ADHD often diagnosed first. Although it was possible the two conditions merely shared some of the same brain pathways, some researchers argued that much of what was diagnosed as ADHD was in fact unrecognized bipolar disorder. An ongoing subject of fierce debate in the psychiatric profession—especially as committees prepare the next version of the *DSM*—concerns whether there is a prodrome to schizophrenia: symptoms that portend later psychosis.

In practice, doctors often hedge their bets. They may tell young patients who are already exhibiting signs of dysfunction that they are "at risk for" developing a more serious condition, such as bipolar disorder or schizophrenia, and that medication will help to lower that risk. "I have had times where I say, 'This is what I think is going on, this is the diagnostic label we use for now,'" says Sherry Goldman, a psychiatrist who treats children, adolescents, and adults in her Rockville, Maryland, practice. "But I also tell them, 'We use labels because we have to, so you get reimbursed by the insurance company, so we can be talking to each other and have some idea what we're talking about.' But I really don't like to pigeon-hole people because they *may* look different years down the road."

The questions of comorbidity, one illness that joins another, and of prodrome, one illness that precedes another, are further complicated by the fact that drugs used to treat one condition may exacerbate or even trigger another. In the 1990s these questions began to take on new urgency as more children and adolescents were treated with medication. With the increase in prescribing since then, these issues are arguably even more pressing now.

Here, the challenge is to distinguish short-term psychiatric side effects from long-term effects that may actually change the course of the illness. For example, a major controversy, discussed in the next chapter, involves kids developing suicidal thoughts or behaviors shortly after beginning antidepressants. But examining the extent to which the drugs increase the risk of suicidal impulses in the short term is very different from asking whether taking an antidepressant when you are ten increases your risk of suicide at twenty. Similarly, stimulants can make kids irritable, impatient, or even depressed when the drug starts to wear off, something that was more common in the 1980s and '90s, before the development of longer-lasting forms of such drugs. That is a different issue from kids with ADHD being prone to developing comorbid conditions like anxiety and depression in the long term. It is less clear whether taking stimulants for ADHD increases the risk of the latter: some animal studies suggest they do, though at least one recent study in kids suggests the opposite.[4]

The relationship between antidepressant treatment and the course of bipolar disorder presents perhaps an even more mind-bending chicken-or-the-egg scenario. Based on observational studies and retrospective interviews of bipolar patients, doctors have known for several decades that bipolar disorder usually first shows up as depression, often in adolescence or early adulthood, and that manic symptoms may not appear until several years later. But they also knew, even before the advent of the SSRIs, that antidepressants could trigger mania in bipolar patients. When the SSRIs came to market in the 1990s, they, like the older drugs, also tended to set off mania in bipolar patients. A single manic episode, or a hypomanic episode combined with a depressive episode, is sufficient for a doctor to diagnose the two main forms of bipolar disorder.[5] But a serious question remains unanswered: can antidepressants prescribed for an initial depression trigger mania *de novo* in young people? Can they, in other words, *cause* someone to have a first manic episode, in a sense producing bipolar illness, usually considered by doctors a serious mental illness that requires a lifetime of medication?

The *DSM*, the go-to book for diagnosis, specifies that a single manic episode caused by an antidepressant is not sufficient for a diagnosis of bipolar disorder, but in practice many psychiatrists consider mania triggered by an antidepressant as a sign that someone is at increased risk for the condition. The researchers Michael Strober and Gabrielle Carlson, some of the first to demonstrate that bipolar disorder could show up in preteens and young teenagers, proposed as early as 1982 that a drug "challenge" might be a way of seeing which youth were headed to a bipolar diagnosis.[6] Today, it remains unclear whether antidepressants can cause a manic episode that would never have occurred otherwise, or whether they uncover a "latent" form of bipolar disorder. As Kiki Chang of UCLA and colleagues put it in a 2010 paper, "The unproven possibility remains that these patients might never have developed manic episodes without this intervention."[7] Meanwhile, top experts say that in the past twenty years the overall course of bipolar disorder has worsened, with the average bipolar adult patient experiencing more rapidly cycling episodes of increasing severity over a lifespan, a phenomenon the journalist Robert Whitaker chronicles in depth in his book *Anatomy of an Epidemic*.[8]

The question of how stimulants affect bipolar disorder is also vexing. There is a high rate of comorbidity between ADHD and bipolar disorder, and it is not unusual for a child diagnosed with the former to be subsequently diagnosed with the latter, as Paul was. But since many children are treated with stimulants before being diagnosed as bipolar, it is not known whether the medications might be affecting the course of the illness. As is the case for antidepressant treatment, stimulants can, rarely, cause short-term psychiatric reactions such as mania and psychosis, but their role in precipitating bipolar disorder remains ambiguous. In one of the most comprehensive studies, which involved kids with a family history of the condition, researchers expected to find a correlation between treatment with antidepressants or stimulants before the initial manic episode and an earlier onset of bipolar disorder. They did not find such a correlation. Instead, the study showed that kids treated with other kinds of medication—a mood stabilizer such as lithium or mood-stabilizing anticonvulsant drugs like Depakote—before they developed mania had their first episode more than three years later, on average, than those who hadn't been medicated previously. The findings suggested that, at least for kids with a family history of the disorder, taking a mood stabilizer might have a protective effect, although it's also possible that they received mood stabilizers in the first place because they were already experiencing more severe symptoms.[9] The findings about mood stabilizers are interesting because, as was apparently the case for Paul, the drugs were used off-label somewhat controversially in the 1990s to treat behavior disorders involving aggression. The drugs could have unpleasant side effects and could even be dangerous—Paul overdosed on his—but conceivably they helped stave off an even earlier onset for kids subsequently diagnosed with bipolar disorder, as Paul was.

Extrapolating the findings about prior antidepressant use by young people like Caleb whose mania shows up later is also difficult. One interesting 2004 study, working from pharmacy claims data from a five-year period, found that compared to peers not taking antidepressants, twice as many young people aged five to twenty-nine experienced bipolar conversion from a diagnosis of anxiety or depression while taking an SSRI antidepressant. Those taking the older tricyclic antidepressants were nearly four times as likely to undergo such a change in diagnosis, as were those taking antidepressants classified as neither SSRIs nor tricyclics. The most vulnerable time seemed to be between ages ten to fourteen when the odds of conversion associated with an antidepressant were one in ten, the researchers found, compared to one in twenty-three among fifteen- to twenty-nine-year-olds.[10]

Unlike some of his peers whom I encountered, including some who attributed panic attacks and other psychiatric symptoms to their medications, Caleb wasn't upset to learn that Zoloft, the same medication that saved him from his crushing depression, may have later sent him spinning out of control. He believed the drug had saved his life. If it had ceased to work, or even propelled him into mania, then so be it; as far as he was concerned, it had done its work. As for Effexor, he'd given it a shot. Knowing the antidepressants alone hadn't tamed his symptoms, he was content to search for another drug that would.

It's important to note that this is Caleb's retrospective analysis of his condition. In the midst of his mania, he wasn't philosophizing about how medication affected him, or analyzing what it *meant* to be bipolar. The same goes for Paul, who was treated with stimulants for years before being diagnosed with bipolar disorder. Paul never took his bipolar diagnosis seriously and in fact was unaware of the link between stimulant treatment and manic episodes, as well as the possible protective role that mood stabilizers, such as the Tegretol he took, may play in staving off mania. So I don't mean to suggest that new symptoms always present a puzzle that young people feel compelled to tackle and solve in the short term. But the ambiguity surrounding their changing condition does in theory present a challenge to adolescents' developing sense of self. For those inclined to introspection and self-definition, this added twist in the plot makes their illness narratives all the more vexed over the long term. Some may have been headed for intractable illness regardless, but the thought that a drug might have set a person on a more serious course that requires additional, heavier-duty medication presents a horrible, haunting "what-if."

James, a young man from California who was diagnosed and medicated with stimulants for ADHD at age five, provides an instructive example. Antidepressants were added to his drug regimen a few years later, as was a diagnosis of conduct disorder and Asperger's, a brand-new diagnosis at the time (it appeared for the first time in the 1994 edition of the *DSM*). Then at twelve he was diagnosed with bipolar disorder and treated with first lithium and then antipsychotics. Was he misdiagnosed with ADHD when all along he was suffering from bipolar disorder? Did he have all of these conditions simultaneously? Did his stimulant treatment, or perhaps his antidepressant treatment, set off his mania, in effect "making" him bipolar? He doesn't himself recall his childhood mood swings, though his parents say he had exhibited them since he was a toddler. For James and so many with comorbid illnesses, each additional disorder, and each additional medication, only multiplies the perplexing variables. Along with the complexities of changing life circumstances, a growing body, and emerging self-awareness, constantly changing symptoms combine to form an infinitely complex calculation. Many children, of course, do not take medication continuously as they mature. Some actively rebel against their medication, but many others get better and go off treatment on their doctor's advice. What, then, does it mean when they run into new problems years later? Should they interpret these symptoms as a recurrence of their previous disorder, or as something altogether new? Do they see their time off medication as a mistake, or as a necessary test period?

Alex, age eighteen
LONG ISLAND, NEW YORK / 2006

Alex's troubles reappeared precisely as he was getting ready to move on, when his life seemed, in some ways, to be taking a turn for the better. He had attended an elite, all-boys' Catholic high school where most of the student body was far wealthier than he, a distinction that dogged him, as he thought the other boys failed to recognize their own privilege and lacked genuine intellectual engagement. He made excellent grades, but was frustrated that, unlike most of his classmates, he had to choose the college that provided the best financial aid package rather than the best education. To save money by living at home, he applied only to schools in the New York area. As it turned out, the best offer came from a private college just a few miles from his old high school, which meant Alex would have to make the same two-hour commute he had made all during senior year, when the family had moved to Brooklyn so that his stepfather could take a job at a real estate office there.

Alex was disappointed to settle for a less prestigious school than he thought his talents and accomplishments merited, but he was optimistic, at least, about the way things were going with his stepfather. Later, with the help of therapy, Alex would classify his stepdad's behavior toward him and his mother as emotionally abusive. For the moment, Alex simply considered him cruel and bullying. The taunts and putdowns subsided toward the end of his senior year, however, when it became clear that he would be putting himself through college with part-time jobs and loans, and therefore didn't pose a financial burden. His stepdad even came to Alex's high school graduation. Then, two weeks later, the spells set in.

For thirty minutes or so, a couple of times a day, Alex felt mired in hopelessness and self-loathing. During the first week of these episodes, he lost ten pounds, too anxious and unhappy to eat. He was working that summer on his former high school's maintenance crew, helping landscape playing fields for the school's grand and expanding campus on Long Island. The property had two baseball fields and was ringed with a line of trees. Alex spent most of his time on the periphery, weeding. He worked alone, which had the advantage of allowing him to fall to pieces when the episodes came on. He would sob in the weeds until he felt strong enough to pull himself together.

The episodes increased throughout the summer until one day Alex counted nine in a single day. He didn't connect these dark, brooding moods to the problems he had had as a ten-year-old when, seemingly out of the blue, he had become obsessed with the thought that he was adopted. Nor did he draw a connection to the fact that he was no longer taking antidepressants. Alex judged himself to have managed fine during the two and a half years since his psychiatrist had him taper off Luvox. Anyway, these episodes felt nothing like his previous worries. Before, he had obsessed over something he knew to be imaginary. After all, he had seen his birth certificate, his hospital bracelet—more than enough proof he was not adopted. This time he felt lonely and desperate in a way that was utterly unfamiliar. He had spent his eighteen years in a mostly self-imposed state of social isolation, content to spend his time alone. Now, he was desperate for social contact, hoping that someone could keep him tethered to the real world.

When he first began worrying at age ten, Alex told his mother immediately. Now, he felt too cut off to alert her. Though his mother wasn't as tuned in to his moods as she once had been, she nevertheless noticed something was wrong. About a month into his mood swings, she suggested maybe he was having a relapse. He had, after all, been diagnosed at age ten with anxiety and depression in addition to OCD, she said. Didn't it seem to Alex that this might be related?

Alex was taken aback. He hadn't known about the diagnoses of anxiety and depression, only the OCD. He had heard his psychiatrist, as well as the therapist he had seen from age ten to twelve, throw the terms around years earlier, yes, but he'd never thought of them as formal diagnoses like his OCD. However, now that his mom laid it out, it did seem to make sense that this breakdown, though far more severe and alarming, might be connected to his previous troubles. It made sense, he reasoned, that anxiety and depression would manifest differently in a ten-year-old than in someone nearly grown-up.

Even when he began to think of his current troubles as likely connected to his past ones, Alex didn't immediately seek help. Being more mature this time around, he thought he ought to be better equipped to shoulder the burden. Moreover, as much as he resented Tony for isolating him from his mom, Alex took some comfort in thinking that Tony's petty, steady abuse had made him, Alex, more independent and self-sufficient. And though he disagreed with Tony about almost everything, Alex had accepted Tony's view that Americans are too quick to medicate away their problems to compensate for inner weakness. He told himself he'd tough it out this time without a pill.

Medical anthropologists talk about the gradual and often quite involved process through which people adopt "illness identities" that, over time, become a fundamental part of their sense of self. Some patients, including psychiatric patients, cling fast to their newfound identities because they provide them with a framework for understanding themselves and the world. But others, regardless of their age or particular demons, eagerly shed their illness identities. When a psychiatric condition first appears in childhood or adolescence and subsequently abates, patients may see themselves not only as recovered, but also as mature adults who have outgrown their troubled, childish selves. To return to illness would be not only to return to an earlier, unhappier time, but, in effect, to regress to a less mature state. "There is this wish and this belief that one simply outgrows the condition and now that one is older and wiser the condition is not going to come back," says Maryland psychiatrist and psychoanalyst Sharon Bisco. "And it can feel like a terrible failure when it does." The doctor's task is to convince the young patient that this is not a failure, not a regression, but merely a common and likely course of a chronic condition.

Believing that one's problems stemmed from a "chemical imbalance" does not necessarily inoculate against feeling like an emotional failure. Chemical problems provoke a psychological response, and most people expect themselves to be better capable of coping as they mature. Alex, for example, concluded that even if the same underlying brain vulnerabilities persisted, he was indeed very different at eighteen than he had been at ten, or at fifteen, when he went off his medication. He wanted to think that he had matured past being the child who ran to his mother at the first sign of trouble. And, as much as he hated his stepfather, Alex had to some extent internalized Tony's ethos of macho independence, which equated pills, and in particular, psychiatric medication, with weakness. Graduating high school and preparing to financially support himself through college, Alex didn't want to be dragged back into a state that was not only characterized by unhappiness and frustration; he thought that a return to psychiatric treatment, and, more specifically, to medication, seemed like a capitulation, like a return to immaturity and powerlessness.

Having begun my own medication treatment at approximately the same age that Alex found himself in danger of needing to resume treatment, I saw things quite oppositely. I associated medication with a newly liberated sense of self. To be more precise, I considered medication an essential means of achieving an independent adult identity. I resisted, therefore, when my hometown pediatrician, who was still writing my prescriptions from afar after I'd gone to college, suggested during my sophomore year that I should see how I fared without Prozac. She was probably following the treatment guidelines of the time, which, as mentioned earlier, recommended a trial end to medication after a single episode of depression had remitted. She didn't mention the guidelines, but discussed my depression as possibly "situational," caused by the stress and frustration of high school, and therefore transient. Now that I was doing well in college, she said, I might do just fine without meds.

Though I tried to act casual, her suggestion surprised and terrified me. Like Elizabeth, who delayed asking to be put back on an antidepressant during her senior year of high school for fear she'd seem weak and drug-dependent, I wanted to appear capable and self-reliant. In truth, however, I considered Prozac my security blanket for adulthood. I was excelling in college, and doing it almost effortlessly. Nothing—absolutely nothing—had been effortless back in high school, before Prozac. I couldn't stand going back to that feeling of trudging—slogging, really—through an oppressive and constricting daily morass.

My doctor suggested tapering off my medication during my college's summer term, when sophomores take classes in an atmosphere that resembles camp as much as it does school. But despite the relative lack of stressors, the experiment nevertheless turned out badly. Within a couple of weeks, I was deteriorating rapidly, unable to focus on my course reading, let alone breeze through it as I once had. Even though I spent many evenings out partying with my friends, I'd find myself feeling isolated in my single dorm room, ruminating about my loneliness and worrying about my deteriorating concentration. In time the rumination gave way to panic.

I was so disturbed by my crumbling sense of stability that I didn't stop to consider how this episode was so *unlike* the state that had led to my going on Prozac two years earlier. In high school I had pushed myself to the limit and maintained a grueling pace that managed simultaneously to bore and exhaust me. This time, with far fewer responsibilities and much lower stakes for the immediate future—no all-important standardized tests, no need of a high GPA since I wasn't applying to grad school—I nevertheless found myself utterly overwhelmed. In high school, I would have treated a course on the philosophy of emotions as a fascinating challenge; not prone to emoting myself, I had always loved a chance to intellectualize and analyze feelings. Now enrolled in such a course, I felt like I was drowning in my own out-of-control emotions, fighting back tears during class and living in a blur of anxiety when I was alone. In high school, social contact, except with my closest friends, had drained me. Now, like Alex, I felt suddenly clingy and needy, so much so that in the course of a ten-week term I managed to go through two different, short-lived relationships. Five or six weeks into the term, I made an appointment at the college health center and, after a therapy appointment with a counselor and then a medication consultation with a psychiatrist, emerged with a new Prozac prescription.

It's striking to me now that I was so blithely confident that it was the same old problem—and that Prozac would work as it had before— despite the unfamiliar symptoms. To my recollection, no one suggested, and I didn't consider, the possibility that what looked like a relapse might be withdrawal, my brain adjusting to functioning without the drug (given that Prozac is one of the antidepressants least likely to cause withdrawal, that seems unlikely, though not impossible). Instead, I took the represcription as confirmation that I did, in fact, have a fundamental, lasting "chemical imbalance" that needed righting. I refused to conceive of this chemical imbalance shifting over time, which is one reason I had considered it absurd of my pediatrician to suggest my depression might no longer require medication treatment. But in assuming so resolutely that I required continuing pharmaceutical treatment, I ended up missing the ways in which my problems—or at least my problems as they manifested themselves—had in fact changed, albeit not as dramatically as Caleb's or Alex's. When, the following summer, I suffered another bout of uncharacteristic, lonely, indecisive nervousness, I brushed it off entirely: this was not depression, at least not in the way I knew it. And I was taking Prozac, so I ought to be just fine. I was therefore unprepared when, a few years later, a spell of anxiety overtook me and quite nearly brought me to my knees.

Looking back, I do recall my high school therapists alluding to the ways in which unresolved anxiety had probably contributed to my eating disorder in ninth and tenth grade. But we hadn't discussed what I was anxious *about*, and somehow, like Alex, I hadn't understood myself as having "an anxiety disorder" *per se*. And although I had read up on eating disorders enough in high school to know that antidepressants could be an effective treatment, I remained unaware of how commonly the drugs were prescribed for anxiety disorders, or how commonly anxiety and depression overlapped. With only one way of understanding my problems, I forced my new symptoms to fit into the same conceptual framework. To do otherwise would have been to dismantle the coherent sense of self I'd worked hard to construct.

As my experience and Alex's illustrate, the way in which doctors or parents explain disorders and the need for medication can have serious consequences when symptoms recur or change at a later stage of development. Whether because of their own uncertainty about the diagnosis, a reluctance to label children, a sense that disorders are too complicated to explain, or skepticism about existing categories of illness, adults often shy away from frank, detailed discussions about the causes of mental disorders, and how medication—and therapy—fit into treating them. I suspect that many adults simply don't realize, or haven't fully processed, how truly disorienting and frightening a changing course of illness can be during adolescence, a time of massive developmental upheaval. Even in the scholarly literature, which is more prone to probing existential questions of this kind than busy clinicians or overwhelmed parents, I found next to nothing examining how the arrival of new diagnoses, new symptoms, or new medications affect the young patient.

Nevertheless, both here and in other contexts, kids do attempt to make sense of their experiences, and they do so with whatever information is available to them. I can't recall where I gleaned the "chemical imbalance" paradigm, but I suspect it was probably from television ads for antidepressants, which had been all over the airwaves since I was in ninth grade. My therapists and pediatrician hadn't defined the source of my problems in any clear way, leaving me to formulate my own, inflexible assessment of my symptoms as chemically induced depression. For a well-read, well-informed teenager, I was nonetheless remarkably ignorant, and remarkably susceptible to the appealing and overly simplified explanations supplied by the drug manufacturers.

Certainly, how much adults ought to explain about the nature of mental illness and medication treatment varies widely from kid to kid, depending on the child's age, and developmental and emotional capacity. Yet, there are certain basic paradigms that kids can grasp. Alex, for example, was able to understand that he took medication to tame his obsessive thoughts and compulsive behaviors, and that he had been diagnosed with a condition called OCD. However, although his psychiatrist and therapist used the terms "depressed" and "anxious," he didn't understand that his medication had also been prescribed to treat clinical depression and anxiety. When symptoms of these conditions came to the fore a few years later, he was unprepared to take them seriously, and as such, he didn't seek professional help until months into his breakdown. Early treatment is supposed to help prevent relapse, not only chemically but also cognitively: educating kids about their conditions can help them understand their symptoms—and themselves—better. And yet, at eighteen, Alex was as completely caught off guard as if he had never been treated at all.

CHAPTER 6

Breakdowns

Caleb, ages nineteen to twenty

TRI-CITIES, WASHINGTON / 2004–2005

Caleb had long comforted himself with thoughts of suicide. In the depressed states that returned every few months after he was treated with Zoloft at thirteen, he had reassured himself that should things grow too intolerable, should this unhappiness become more than a temporary blip, he could always end it. In these states, he rehearsed his old, familiar suicide plans incessantly, considering logistics, and weighing pros and cons. The plans seemed to have formed grooves in his brain, well-worn paths he could follow almost automatically, he knew them so well. With the advent of mania toward the end of high school, these reflective, suicidal musings disappeared. In his most elevated moods Caleb felt invincible. But in his mixed states, when his anxiety, depression, and mania produced a horrible cocktail of agitated desperation, he wanted to escape from himself, not mull over the means of escape. It was in one of these intolerable mixed states when, unable to calm down merely by contemplating killing himself, he decided, finally, to go ahead and do it.

Caleb had grown up boating and playing in the Columbia River, which flows south from the Canadian Rockies and forms much of the border between Washington State and Oregon before emptying into the Pacific. Around two in the morning one day in early spring, a few months after he began taking the atypical antipsychotic drug Zyprexa to soothe his delusions and paranoia, Caleb was not inclined to ponder his options. His thoughts settled in the first groove available to him, and that happened to be jumping off the "blue bridge," which he judged to be the highest of the three grand bridges connecting the cities of Pasco and Kennewick, Washington.

Caleb's psychiatrist had once said, "If you ever feel like you're going to kill yourself, by all means call this number first," and had pressed into his hand a card bearing the number of a suicide hotline. Now, suddenly, Caleb remembered the wallet-sized card, and for reasons he later couldn't explain, he fished it out and dialed the hotline. A girl picked up, sounding perky and clueless and no older than he. She told him not to despair; there was help—therapy and medications that could fix his problems. "I've been in counseling," Caleb told her angrily, thinking back to his time in cognitive-behavioral therapy years earlier. "I've been on medication for years. I don't think you should be telling me what to do." He was furious that someone who knew nothing about him or his particular demons would presume to judge his life worth living. In a blind rage, he hung up the phone, got in his car, and began driving. *Let's go*, he thought. *If the cops start chasing me, we're going for a ride.*

The bridge, nearly fifteen miles from Caleb's home, was topped with a giant American flag that at nighttime was lit up like a beacon. He could see it from a mile away, looming larger as he approached. To the east was a suspension bridge, its cables bathed in golden light. On the opposite bank, some cop cars were parked, lights flashing. Caleb didn't know it, but the suicide hotline had tracked his number and alerted the police, who had rushed to his parents' house and pounded on the door. When they found he had already left, the department issued an all points bulletin instructing law enforcement to close off the bridges.

At the moment, however, the cops were just waiting on the opposite bank. They didn't seem inclined to stop him, so Caleb parked his car on the bridge and hopped over the chest-high metal barrier onto a little walkway for maintenance workers. He peered over the edge at the dark water, which wasn't as far down as he had imagined. Having learned in his physics class to calculate the height of a structure based on how long it takes for an object to fall, Caleb pulled a pack of gum from his pocket and tossed one stick after another, counting off the seconds before each piece hit the water. By his rough calculations, the bridge wasn't more than eighty or a hundred feet high.

Caleb had done some recreational jumping from cliffs and bridges in his time, and it occurred to him that eighty feet wasn't very high. Jumping from the Golden Gate Bridge killed nearly everyone, but it was much taller—250 feet. Caleb's psychiatrist had, in fact, treated one of the rare people who survived that jump. He told Caleb that the instant this man stepped off, all his anxiety disappeared, and he regretted his decision. But Caleb wasn't thinking about that regretful jumper right now. He was gazing down into the black water, and thinking how frigid it would be at this time of year. It was glacier water from the mountains. What if he jumped and got caught in the tangle of steel reinforcements at the bridge's base? What if the strong current sucked him under? Drowning seemed to him a particularly unpleasant way to go. Or what if he got pulled out at the last minute with brain damage from lack of oxygen or legs that had to be amputated from the freezing temperatures? At the moment, the idea of being trapped in a hospital bed indefinitely, unable to move, frightened him more than anything. He backed away a little from the edge and walked slowly back to his car to think some more.

During his agitated, mixed state of the past few weeks, Caleb had come to consider it something of a miracle that he had survived this long. Now, as his twentieth birthday approached, it occurred to him that he been severely suicidal at age twelve and that those impulses had returned approximately every three months since. Before his bipolar disorder had shown up, he had considered antidepressant medication at once something that he absolutely required to stay alive and also something that might not necessarily save him from killing himself. As his manias had set in and he had grown paranoid, even delusional, he had become convinced that his parents bitterly resented his living in their house and wanted him to move out. The very thought of becoming a homeless person living on the streets made him worry obsessively about what would happen if he couldn't pay for his prescriptions. Now, that seemed immaterial. Medication, it seemed, had done nothing but stave off the inevitable for eight long years.

Caleb did not jump from the bridge. While he sat in his car, a strange calm came over him, and he ceased to feel anything. A fireman knocked on the window and asked how he was doing. Caleb, impassive, said he was doing okay. And then the assembled cops were bundling him into a cruiser and driving him to the county's emergency psychiatric facility. Caleb cooperated fully, and the authorities concluded that once he had stepped away from the edge, he was no longer an acute danger to himself or others; therefore, he didn't have to be forcibly hospitalized or medicated. As he sat alone in a half-lit reception area waiting for his parents to arrive and take him home, Caleb felt numb. This time, unlike in middle school, he didn't feel enlightened or profound or special. He simply felt nothing at all. Caleb's near-suicide had been altogether impulsive, but it was the culmination of more than two years of unchecked mania and mixed manic-depressive states that had shaken him to his core.

A suicide attempt, or even a close call like Caleb's, is one of the most dramatic manifestations of what are colloquially referred to as breakdowns. Even though the term has no specific diagnostic meaning, it is deeply embedded in our cultural vocabulary—a shorthand for acute psychiatric crises that seriously affect day-to-day functioning, causing heightened or unmanageable levels of distress, and precipitating a loss of self.

A breakdown is devastating because one realizes "that there is no self that will not crumble," as Andrew Solomon writes in *The Noonday Demon*, his "atlas of depression."[1] Yet, as Solomon explains, depressive breakdowns are fundamentally atemporal, and I think the same may be said of any acute psychiatric episode. During the breakdown itself, you are enmeshed in an inescapable present. You are not systematically considering the reasons for your deterioration, nor pondering the role of medication, past, present, or future. But eventually, after the moment of crisis recedes, you must make sense of what happened.

A person's stage in life and his treatment history shape how he integrates the breakdown into what medical anthropology calls an "illness narrative." A person's age at the first acute crisis shapes the conclusions he draws, both in the moment and long afterward, about how medication factored in, and what to do about it. Yet there is little research comparing breakdowns in childhood with those in adolescence, midlife, or old age, and scant attention to how people strive to comprehend breakdowns that occur when they have a history of medication treatment, versus those that occur when people are, as clinicians put it, "treatment-naive."

For earlier generations who grew up before psychiatric medication became so widespread, it often took a complete breakdown, typically well into adulthood, before one received any kind of treatment. Older people face the challenge of accepting and understanding a new illness identity in which their problems have boiled over rather than simmered beneath the surface. The illness narrative takes a very different shape for the current generation of young adults who were diagnosed and treated with medication at a young age. If their pills work well, their illness identity may well have faded into the background. But medications, although they can prevent relapses and breakdowns, aren't guaranteed to work forever. The first major breakdown, then, will pose a major new challenge: how to understand an unprecedented or recurrent collapse as part of an ongoing narrative of dysfunction and treatment. Even more than the appearance of new symptoms and diagnoses (discussed in chapter 5), for many young people, a full-on breakdown with a serious loss of day-to-day functioning is profoundly disturbing. After you have spent years on drugs and have integrated them into your life and identity, a breakdown is a sobering indication that you aren't fixed after all.

When medication fails, despite supposedly being a safety net to keep you from bottoming out, you may begin to think, as Caleb did, that medication merely postponed the inevitable. Through years of living with depression, Caleb had maintained a clear line in his mind between sane people like himself and those he judged insane—the crazy guys on the street corner mumbling to themselves or shouting incoherent warnings of impending doom, the son of a family friend with bipolar disorder who heard voices and conversed with imaginary companions.

When Caleb was in high school, the boy had told him that he tried hard to ignore the voices when he was in public settings because, although he believed they were real, he knew better than to betray his delusions to others. Now that Caleb had lived through his own delusions, such as the conviction that his parents didn't love him and preferred him to move out and live on the streets, the line between sanity and insanity seemed anything but clear. Nor were medications a guarantee of staying on the "sane" side. Zoloft, mostly prescribed for people who were not psychotic or delusional, had launched him into mania. Zyprexa, the atypical antipsychotic he had been taking for a few months to control his mania, had not prevented steps toward suicide. Caleb now suspected it may have clouded his thinking, thereby contributing to his impulsive decision. It was time to try something new. Caleb's psychiatrist prescribed Depakote, an antiseizure drug used to modulate depression and mania. Even after finding a tolerable dose, which took months of calibration, Caleb was left with the difficult work of parsing what had happened to him and determining how he ought to go on.

Caleb's quarterly sessions with his psychiatrist were primarily intended to monitor his response to the new medication, but after the incident at the bridge his doctor tried to delve a little into the circumstances of Caleb's life. Caleb belonged to a "fight club" modeled after the 1999 Brad Pitt and Edward Norton movie by that name, which, according to *Maxim* magazine, was "commonly credited with setting off the trend for semi-organized underground slugfests among teenage boys and young men."[2] Caleb was joking around with the doctor about this fight club, being charming and generally putting on a good performance, when his psychiatrist asked what, exactly, he had been feeling in the midst of his last fight.

Caleb couldn't answer. As the doctor stared at him, he sat there paralyzed, jaw clenched, emotions coursing through his body like an electric current. He thought about how on that night, during the last fight, he did not feel like himself at all. He might as well have been watching Ed Norton throw the punches. Now, the emotions he ought to have been feeling during the fight and, indeed, all the emotions he hadn't felt for months suddenly flooded over him. He sat there making soft, nervous braying noises. It seemed like ages before he could bring himself to form words.

Research on suicide and suicide attempts suggest that people usually enter something of a trance that, if they survive, can leave them feeling disconnected from their emotions and the world for weeks, months, or even years. But even before the attempt, Caleb had at times felt alienated from his feelings, removed from his own body. To him, the mania resembled the feeling he'd had as a little boy when his father tossed him in the air—thrilled up until a point, and then, when he soared just a little too high, terrified. Now, the simple question that began nearly every conversation—"How are you?"—left him mutely fumbling for a response.

A few months after he nearly leaped from the bridge, Caleb and his father began planning a trip to Europe with some of his dad's frequent-flier miles. Somewhere in his chain of online meanderings, Caleb had discovered that the pharmaceutical giant Pfizer, which had developed Zoloft, had a clinical trials laboratory in Belgium, not too far from the World War II battlefields he and his dad would be visiting. He told his dad he wanted to see where Pfizer manufactured the drug that he credited with saving his life at age thirteen. On the standard visitors' tour, Caleb was ushered into an area where the scientists were at work. A beautiful female doctor greeted them. In her white coat she looked almost angelic to Caleb. Overcome with emotion, he shook her hand and said, "I just want to tell you that you saved my life. I really want to thank you." She smiled and said, with a slight French accent, "That's wonderful—I'm so happy you feel that way. A lot of people are very angry at us, you know. They want to sue us!" Caleb was shocked. Here was this angelic woman doing good work. To think how many lives antidepressants had saved, how much crime they had prevented, how many families they had kept intact—it boggled his mind that people didn't appreciate that.

It was the summer of 2004, and back in the United States, specially convened FDA committees were deliberating over troubling data that had emerged regarding young people and SSRIs. The FDA had already issued two recent public health advisories warning of a link between antidepressants and suicide; now, a meta-analysis of studies showed that SSRIs doubled the risk of suicidal thinking and behavior in depressed adolescents from 2 percent to 4 percent, almost always in the weeks after treatment began. The data in question did not include any completed suicides, but that fall, the FDA mandated a "black box" suicide warning for pediatric prescriptions; two years later, despite several well-regarded analyses contesting the agency's conclusions, it would extend the warning to include prescriptions for young adults twenty-four and younger.

Caleb had heard nothing of the controversy. But in any case, he later concluded the subject didn't apply to him. He couldn't remember if at the time of his near-suicide he had been taking Paxil, an SSRI. It seemed more likely to him that the doctor added Paxil after his suicide attempt, as one of several medication changes. Either way, he insisted that Paxil hadn't spurred him to action. If anything, he thought, Zyprexa was to blame, because it further clouded his already distorted thinking, which included a bizarre, subconscious conviction that he would not make it to age twenty (the attempt occurred a week before his twentieth birthday, a connection he only made later). As for the charge that SSRIs did more net harm than good for depressed teens, he didn't consider it relevant to his experience. In his mind, Zoloft, his antidepressant through middle and high school, retained its original perfection. The drug had saved Caleb when he was a suicidal middle schooler.

There is something magical about one's first medication—if one has a quick and positive response, as both Caleb and I did. Since Caleb's adolescent depression was far more severe than mine, I can only imagine how redemptive his recovery on Zoloft must have seemed to him. He venerated the drug for allowing him to experience the carefree life of an ordinary teenager, at least when he wasn't having one of his periodic bouts of hopelessness or a panic attack triggered by his fear of crowds. (Football games and pep rallies, for example, brought flashbacks of the brutal bullying he had suffered in middle school.) This time, though, Caleb's recovery was a slow process, aided but not instantly resolved by medication.

Though he later insisted he wasn't angry or bitter about Effexor, which he had taken a couple of years earlier, spinning him further into possible mania, or about Zyprexa failing to diffuse his agonizing mixed states, or about Depakote working so subtly and so slowly, Caleb's pilgrimage to the Pfizer research lab in Belgium bore witness to his nostalgia about his previous miraculous recovery. This time, it took months before Depakote began to feel like a pair of strong hands that scooped him up at a fragile moment and set him back on reasonably solid ground. Instead of going out and dancing manically until dawn, he found himself content to stay in on Friday nights. As if stunned by the drama of all he'd been through, he wanted the dullest, most ordinary life possible. His mood stabilizers might have played a role, but the change was so gradual that it seemed to him then that this need for serenity represented as much a natural desire to recalibrate, having seen the highest highs and the lowest lows, as it did a change brought about by drugs. Indeed, six months after the episode on the bridge and several months after the trip to Belgium, very much in need of concrete reassurance, he got a tattoo on his upper back. In thick, gothic letters it paraphrased an old Russian peasant saying: The pain of today will be gone tomorrow.

In 1995, Kay Redfield Jamison, a Johns Hopkins University psychiatrist and coauthor of the classic textbook on bipolar disorder, became one of the first clinician-researchers to go public with her illness. Her book *An Unquiet Mind*, an arresting and lyrical account of her own struggle with manic depression, describes her dilatory adherence to lithium and the resulting eighteen-month suicidal depression. That episode culminated in her decision to use the instrument of her treatment as the means of her own destruction, "a solution," she writes, "that seemed to me to be poetic in its full-circledness."[3] Even though lithium is highly toxic in even slightly elevated doses, Jamison survived a massive overdose, and remained on the drug because at the time, in the mid-1970s, it was by far the most effective treatment available to control cycling manias and depressions. Jamison's memoir strives to reconcile her image of the "dreary, crabbed, pained woman who desperately wished only for death and took a lethal dose of lithium to accomplish it" with her earlier image of herself as an enthusiastic, ambitious, and energetic young woman.[4] How could someone who had been so in love with life, she asks, so fervently desire death? And, I myself wondered, how was she to recover not only her zest for life but also her faith in a medication that had let her down and very nearly killed her?

As many other narratives of severe mental illness, especially schizophrenia, attest, this is a difficult and grim lesson, often learned only after repeated and dramatic breakdowns. But at least these situations have the advantage of lacking ambiguity: someone fails to take her antipsychotic drugs, and ends up floridly psychotic; someone fails to take his mood stabilizer, falls into a suicidal depression, and nearly ends his life. Suffering a breakdown while on medication doesn't offer this conceptual leg up: recovery involves not just the work of rebuilding one's sense of self, but of figuring out how to approach one's treatment.

One advantage of getting treatment relatively early in life is that it gives you a head start on understanding these issues. Recoveries are never easy, but the benefit of experience often makes them easier. The transitions and change inherent in adolescence and young adulthood, not to mention the instability of diagnoses, symptoms, and treatment over time, complicate recovery. People medicated from a young age aren't likely to suffer a single, serious episode and then, presto, with a quick change of medication, be set for life. A breakdown is a lesson that they cannot overcome their problems as easily as they may have thought. As Claire's father, a psychologist and patient activist who is schizophrenic himself, wrote in an article, "Recovery is best understood as a process, not an outcome."[5] Claire suffered two dramatic breakdowns, one in college and one immediately afterward, but she was able to see them as more severe versions of the relapses she'd suffered since going on medication at age eleven. A drug would stop working, her depression would reappear, and she would need to switch to a new drug. To her a breakdown was a sign that she needed to monitor herself more carefully, and to intervene before her depression overwhelmed her.

Many of Claire's peers adopted a similarly utilitarian approach. Others were far less sure how to proceed. If you experienced a dramatic turnaround on a particular medication only to suffer a breakdown later, as I did, recovery involves coming to terms with having a condition that requires more than a one-time biochemical tweak. If you've spent much of your childhood and adolescence looking, without success, for a drug that offers relief, a collapse means coming up with reasons to keep looking—or putting your faith in another treatment altogether. In the midst of a crisis, some young people feel that they need something more. When Alex, who had been treated with the antidepressant Luvox for OCD, depression, and generalized anxiety, had a breakdown several years after going off the medication midway through high school, returning to his old medical regimen seemed insufficient. Although he actively lobbied for hospitalization, new treatment protocols and insurance limits made that difficult.

Alex, ages eighteen to nineteen
BROOKLYN, NEW YORK / 2006–2007

Alex had tried to check himself into a psychiatric unit a few months after his depressive episodes set in, having realized the failure of his medication cocktail: short-acting anxiety drugs and Luvox, now at one-fifth the dose he had taken as a child. Alex thought the antidepressant dosing absurd, and resented his new psychiatrist's refusal to consider his opinion on the matter. Since neither his psychiatrist nor his therapist seemed to register quite how far gone he was, he thought inpatient treatment might be the only way to rout the anguish and to get someone to take his condition seriously. But when he enlisted his mother, a nurse, to help him check into a psych unit nearby, the admitting staff turned him away because he had no immediate plan to kill himself.

Back home, Alex reflected bitterly on his situation. He considered himself someone with a reasonably well-established history of psychiatric problems, someone who knew himself well and was, even in his compromised state of mind, a logical and careful decision maker (he did not consider that just a few months earlier he had been completely convinced he could make the breakdown go away with mere resolve). It infuriated him that the professionals weren't taking seriously his pleas for help. Without some drastic intervention, he was convinced he would only get worse.

Sure enough, at Christmas dinner, Alex and his stepfather clashed again. His stepdad claimed Alex's moodiness was just jealousy about

Tony coming between Alex and his mother. "Ugh," Alex said. "Isn't that, like, totally Oedipal?" Alex's mom quickly moved to smooth things over—she had a feeling Tony wouldn't understand what "Oedipal" meant, which would make him even angrier. But Alex felt himself slipping into the dark. The next day, he insisted that his mother and stepdad bring him to a different hospital. This time, when the psychiatric nurses asked if he planned to kill himself, he lied and said he did.

The hospitalization lasted only four days, but it did what Alex had hoped. Seeing other, more disturbed patients helped him get a grip on his situation. He also got a more powerful medication, the atypical antipsychotic Risperdal, which is often given to sedate agitated patients in inpatient settings. The first powerful dose made him slur his words as thoughts careened in loops through his head. The next night the nurses administered a smaller dose, and Alex awoke to find his head clearer than it had been in years, certainly since before his stepfather filled the house with conflict. Suddenly the world seemed like a softer and gentler, less cruel and arbitrary place. The future might have something to offer him after all.

Had Alex been born even one or two decades earlier, he might well have had an easier time getting admitted to a psychiatric ward in the first place and would likely have stayed much longer, perhaps for weeks, or even months. Alex's mother happened to have an excellent insurance plan, but the structural changes in the way insurance reimbursed hospitals had already created a large-scale shift in the way inpatient units operated. In the 1970s and 1980s, even as public adult psychiatric wards were emptying out, there had been a boom in private inpatient treatment for adolescents.[6] New private wards opened, admissions went up, and the mean length of stay increased relative to that of adults.[7] But with the rapid advent of managed care in the late 1980s and early 1990s, private insurance companies adopted aggressive cost-cutting measures, which encouraged outpatient treatment over more expensive inpatient admissions. These measures made it more difficult to be admitted in the first place and capped the length of stay, which had declined to an average pediatric stay of ten days in 2001, down from more than forty in 1988.[8] Four-day admissions like Alex's became common.

The new restrictions made sense in many ways: of all treatments, hospitalization had the least evidence of positive outcomes for young people. Lasting for months or even years, it could suck up key developmental portions of a young person's life, a sentiment encapsulated by the title of Susanna Kaysen's best-selling 1993 memoir of her teenage hospitalization during the 1960s: *Girl, Interrupted.*

Restrictions on admissions and shorter lengths of stay, however, created their own problems. As public wards closed, beds for both children and adults were in short supply, which could make it quite difficult, as Alex found, to gain admittance. And, because many private insurance plans began to require medication initiation as a condition of reimbursing even a short stay, doctors faced increased pressure to throw some medication—any medication—at their patients. The problem was that most young people were already on a cocktail of drugs when they arrived. As Gabrielle Carlson, a pioneer in the diagnosis of youth bipolar disorder and the director of child and adolescent psychiatry at Stony Brook University Medical Center in Long Island, explains, short stays allow no time to establish a medication-free baseline before making a treatment decision. Instead, doctors work with the cards they are dealt. Alex, for example, entered the hospital taking a low dose of the antidepressant Luvox. Doctors gave him Risperdal, a fast-acting antipsychotic, to calm him down, and upped the dosage of Luvox to the level he had taken as a kid. Since Luvox is a slow-acting drug, there was no time to see how he fared before he had to be released.

Alex had not, in fact, wanted a long hospital stay, and upon release, he was optimistic, encouraged by his doctors' observation that he was remarkably lucid compared to the ward's other patients. But a short-term improvement in the hospital doesn't always mean a breakdown is over. Many patients end up being readmitted; several studies have shown a correlation between declining lengths of stay in the 1990s and rising rates of readmission for both adults and children.[9] Just a few days after being released, Alex deteriorated when his stepfather's hostility made him realize that nothing had changed.

Alex's mood lifted as spring-term college courses approached, but then one Saturday around noon, as he lazed about, watching TV in his room, he heard his mom and stepfather arguing again—something about money. As their voices grew angrier, his mood plunged and he was flooded with hopelessness. Even after all Alex had been through, his mom was still with his stepfather, and Alex was still living in the shadow of their dysfunctional, fraught relationship. He couldn't see the point in putting up with it any longer. Three weeks after feigning suicidal intentions to get help, Alex decided to kill himself—and to do it in the very manner he had described in his lie to the admitting nurse: throwing himself in front of a subway on the above-ground tracks near his mother's house.

Having made the decision, he felt strangely elated, liberated, and lightened of his load, a feeling that many depressed people report experiencing once they have made the decision to end it all. While his mom and stepdad continued to argue, Alex slipped out of the apartment into the cold and began the two-mile trek to the subway.

In the end, like Caleb, Alex didn't kill himself. Although he had not intended his action as a cry for help, it served that purpose: he called his aunt right before he stepped onto the tracks. She patched his mother into a conference call, and together they talked him out of it. His mother didn't take his plan as seriously as he thought she should have. Instead, she yelled at him for causing a scene and drove him straight to his evening job at an office-cleaning janitorial service. Still, he had managed to make it clear in numerous ways, to himself and others, how desperate he felt, and that had its own value, somehow. Just standing there near the tracks had cleared his head, shocked him back into his regular, logical frame of mind, much as the hospitalization and the Risperdal had done. He felt lucid enough that he didn't want to return to the hospital. Nor did his psychiatrist adjust his medication again for many months. Instead, Alex began the slow process of building himself back up again.

Alex and Caleb were both living at home when they reached their respective crisis points, and Claire, when she had a breakdown in college, was near enough for her mother to arrive on the scene in relatively short order. Though Alex had a strained relationship with his mother, a very poor one with his stepfather, and an indifferent and slightly hostile one with both his therapist and psychiatrist of four months, he still found some comfort in having his breakdown on familiar territory. For people who move away from home before experiencing a crisis, the combination of new surroundings, the lack of a family support network, and the allure of starting out afresh on one's own make securing help all the more difficult.

For those in college, there is usually a student health center that can be utilized in a crisis, even if it is understaffed or doesn't have psychiatric experts available. For those not in college, there is often a serious gap in care. A 2008 report by the Government Accountability Office (GAO) estimated that 2.4 million young adults aged eighteen to twenty-four have a serious mental illness—defined as having during the past twelve months a diagnosis of psychosis or bipolar disorder, a serious suicide attempt, or any other disorder that seriously impaired functioning for at least thirty days in the past year. The GAO reported significant challenges transitioning from pediatric to adult care, and highlighted the particular difficulty of doing so for those suffering from acute mental illness, especially since states' clinical criteria for providing public mental health care and disability benefits are stricter for adults than for children.[10]

Even ready access to campus care is no guarantee of prompt intervention in the event of a breakdown. College counseling centers are overwhelmed with an influx of students requesting help, especially since there has been such a dramatic increase in those who have been diagnosed and treated with medication prior to entering college.[11] Counseling center staff speculate that the increased burden is, somewhat paradoxically, due to more people being diagnosed and treated at young ages, since widespread early intervention enables college enrollment by students who in an earlier era might have been sidelined by psychiatric troubles. A report on the University of California system's mental health services found, for example, that one in four students who sought help at campus counseling centers was already taking psychotropic medication—and that didn't count the many students who took meds but didn't go to the counseling center.[12]

Many of these students had, like Elizabeth, been sufficiently stabilized to survive high-pressure high schools and to meet their parents' demanding expectations; yet simply making it to college isn't enough.[13] Students whose mental health is already somewhat tenuous upon arrival must find a way to thrive, or at least survive, in an environment that can present greater psychological, intellectual, and social challenges than life at home. It isn't clear, moreover, what role universities ought to play in accommodating this wave of troubled students. The student movements of the 1960s effectively terminated the tradition of the university acting *in loco parentis*—monitoring and intervening in students' private lives. But in the late 1990s and early 2000s, several high-profile student suicides—and subsequent parental lawsuits—had colleges scrambling to reevaluate their hands-off strategies. Universities often found themselves caught between parents who demanded closer scrutiny and students who resisted institutional incursions. As the director of Harvard's counseling center pointed out in a 2004 book aimed at parents, colleges' mental health services have no way of identifying the substantial population of students with a pre-college history of medication, since matriculating students often do not report their existing mental health problems in the hope of making a fresh start.[14]

So long as everything is going well, students might be fine having their hometown doctors calling in medication refills. But when things start to go badly, these students find themselves in a bind, since many doctors hesitate to change medication or dosages for a patient they are no longer seeing regularly. Since college counseling centers generally do not have access to a student's previous psychiatric records, and since recounting one's symptoms and prescriptions afresh is tedious and exhausting even in the best of times, approaching or experiencing a breakdown at college can be downright terrifying.

Elizabeth, ages eighteen to twenty-two
WASHINGTON, DC, SUBURBS AND
SOUTHERN CALIFORNIA / 1999–2003
Elizabeth entered her prestigious liberal arts college as one of the many medicated kids seeking a fresh start. She was hopeful that the sunny,

laid-back atmosphere of southern California would enable her to leave behind her checkered academic record and to escape the continuing tensions between her parents, who were now in a long-term separation. After four years, she had made peace with taking both an antidepressant to improve her mood and a stimulant to counter her ADHD. But she had a rocky freshman year, making few close friends, and experiencing severe anxiety over academics that left her paralyzed and shaking late at night, unable to complete assignments. The summer after her freshman year, she had to contend with her father going into rehab for alcoholism and indications that her sister was an alcoholic as well.

A few weeks into her sophomore year, she ran out of Celexa, the SSRI antidepressant prescribed by her psychiatrist at home. Preoccupied with her social life, anxious about academics, and overwhelmed by the difficulty of getting her mother's insurance to pay for an out-of-state refill, she did nothing. Shortly thereafter, she went five days without sleeping. On the fifth day, she took a Spanish test in a bleary-eyed stupor, without having studied a whit. When, to her horror, she got a D, she felt so alarmed and exhausted that she flew back to DC for a short fall break and spent the next few days sleeping almost nonstop.

Back on campus after break, Liz confided in two friends that she was so depressed and agitated she was tempted to cut herself to relieve some of the tension, as she had done in high school after going off her Prozac. One friend insisted on inspecting Liz's arms every day to make sure she hadn't hurt herself. Liz found it strangely comforting that he cared enough to do such a thing. The other friend, who was bipolar and on medication, thought that Liz's five days without sleep was evidence of a manic episode, and that she'd now entered a depressive phase. He considered her situation serious enough to require immediate intervention. Liz countered that her ADHD was simply messing with her focus, as always, and that the depression that had plagued her since preadolescence had merely returned to sap her motivation. Giving up her antidepressants so suddenly that fall had been a bad idea, she told him; now that she'd secured a refill, she'd be all right. He disagreed and urged her to seek counseling and perhaps a change in medication. She declined. When he threatened to go to the dean, she stopped speaking to him.

This episode, alarming in itself, set a pattern for the long, slow unraveling that would play out over the next two and a half years, culminating in Liz failing out of college and moving back to her mother's house. Like so much else in her experience of illness, the breakdown was hard for Liz to demarcate and define. During a yearlong mandated academic leave of absence precipitated by failing grades, she felt she was going insane—slowly, agonizingly slowly, as though bits of her were flaking off and disappearing into the ether. The gradual deterioration was maddening. The drugs—Celexa and later Zoloft to counter her depression, the sedative-hypnotic drug Ambien to help her sleep, the stimulant Dexedrine to give her energy and help her focus, and the short-acting antianxiety drug Klonopin to quell the worst of her panic—kept her from truly bottoming out, but she wondered if the drugs were really giving her a shot at recovery, or whether all the pharmaceutical tinkering was only leaving her in a horrible limbo. Without a dramatic, obvious breakdown that couldn't be ignored, she didn't see how she could make the people around her understand how far gone she really was.

Even her most dramatic period of dysfunction to date was in some ways a partial and private breakdown, not a total collapse. She had returned to campus after failing many courses and a yearlong leave of absence, which she spent back home in Maryland, adjusting her medications, finally entering semi-regular therapy, and taking some community college courses to try to make up credits. That spring, she continued to fiddle with her medications, finally relenting and seeing someone at the campus health center. As she failed to complete assignments and fell further and further behind, however, her panic spiraled. To deal with the mounting tension, she began cutting herself again, late at night, when the Klonopin and Ambien failed to calm her sufficiently. Whereas during sophomore year she had talked to friends about her urge to cut, this time she restricted her accounts to the occasional blocked, private entry in an online diary. It was the spring of 2003, and she had noticed cutting in the news a lot recently. It seemed unbelievably clichéd, the desperation of a sixteen-year-old girl—the sort of thing, in fact, she had herself done as a sixteen-year-old girl. And not to have gotten past it by now, even when she was on a cocktail of four different drugs, was mortifying. She was regressing. With a little over a week left to turn in her papers, she went to the mall and stole a pair of rainbow shoelaces, something she would have been too levelheaded to attempt even back in middle school. At the end of the month, she received word that she had failed out of school for good. Back home, she was left to figure out what had happened and how to pick up the pieces.

Whatever the circumstances, a breakdown requires explaining. In our culture, personal and professional success depend on being able to make a case for yourself, to put your life into a coherent and convincing story, to present a résumé without suspicious gaps. Having an illness show up for the first time in early adulthood is terribly difficult in itself, but if the medications work, they provide a ready-made story: "I started having some problems, but I got some medications, and now I'm doing better." If one has a breakdown after having already spent one's formative years on medication, explanations are harder, both to oneself and to others. The looming question is: Why don't you have it figured out by now?

Liz had been taking a variety of meds in different combinations for eight long years, and still hadn't found a way to stay calm and focused enough to complete the work college demanded. To what extent this was a failure of will, a failure of upbringing, a failure of biology, or a failure of medical science, she just couldn't say. But this ambivalence was not, she reflected in a message to a friend, what people wanted to hear. They wanted you to say that you'd been having some problems, but that you'd finally gotten some meds, or some therapy, or both, and were now doing better. Since she could neither tell that story nor explain what had happened, she simply cut off contact with her college friends.

Failing out did have the rather grim advantage of making her, as well as her doctors and parents, take her anxiety more seriously. Her flameout was a rebuke to her abilities, but also a validation of her disabilities. It gave her a reason to get serious about her mental health care in the same way that being forced to take a leave of absence from school eighteen months earlier had motivated her to see both a therapist and a psychiatrist regularly. Though she had let herself run out of Zoloft, her latest antidepressant, during her final, panicked weeks at school, when she returned home she got a refill, procured more Klonopin, and made arrangements to switch to a new stimulant drug for ADHD, in hopes it would cause less nausea and that she'd therefore be more inclined to take it regularly. And she geared up, quite optimistically, for a summer term of courses at a college in Colorado, something she'd signed up for before failing out, but which would at least be good for some college credits.

The summer term started well but ended with her failing to turn in the final paper for a key class. That fall, back at her mother's house in DC and in the process of applying for transfer admission to several colleges, she hit a wall, unable to craft any kind of plausible story about her spotty academic past. One bad semester she would have had no trouble explaining; one bad year she could have finessed (indeed, she had successfully explained it a year earlier when she had to petition the deans to readmit her after her forced leave of absence). Even having failed out of one school but having done very well in Colorado could have provided a story of redemption. But having screwed up twice, at two different schools, in similar ways, defied any acceptable explanation. It would have been so much simpler if she could tell a slightly different version of her story, if she could truthfully say that although she had been diagnosed with depression and ADHD as a young teenager, she had more recently suffered a couple of manic episodes, had been diagnosed with bipolar disorder, but was now on medication and doing fine! But her problems, and her response to meds, remained maddeningly nebulous. Both she and her psychiatrist thought she might have had a manic episode during the fall of her sophomore year, when she didn't sleep for five days, and that she could possibly have had a second one during her last semester at college. But the doctor considered her history too irregular to give her a diagnosis of bipolar disorder. It wasn't clear, for example, whether the initial, supposed manic episode was caused by too high a dose of stimulants, by her switch from one antidepressant to another a few weeks beforehand, or by her having run out of her antidepressant for a few days. Besides, the fact remained that she was on medications, a raft of them, and had succumbed nonetheless. How was she to convince an admissions office that she could ever manage to get the drugs right, that she would successfully find some elusive mix of energy, motivation, calm, and poise that the meds had thus far failed to provide?

The impossibility of the task so exacerbated her anxiety that she didn't apply to a new college that year after all. It also colored her attitude toward her medication treatment. Since she wasn't in school, there seemed no reason to take stimulants. Then, she let herself run out of Klonopin and Zoloft. There no longer seemed any point in bothering.

Over the next few years, as she sought to complete her degree at several different schools, Liz continued to have the same problems justifying and packaging herself. She also continued to have a fraught, on-again, off-again record of adhering to her meds, and the inconsistency only made her story harder to tell. She had grown up with nearly every material advantage, successful parents, high intelligence, prestigious schooling, and top-notch psychiatric treatment. Yes, her parents had a troubled marriage and her father and sister struggled with alcoholism, but it wasn't as though Liz had suffered a psychotic break, or been diagnosed with some devastating physical debility, or lost a close relative. If she had failed to attend therapy or adhere to her medications, she was hard-pressed to find anyone to blame but herself.

Both Alex and Liz went through their initial years of treatment without taking their conditions very seriously. Alex responded well to his first antidepressant, so well in fact that his doctor discontinued his prescription after a few years. When Alex did fine without it, he concluded that he'd been an "overmedicated kid." Liz also didn't consider her problems to be particularly severe compared to kids she knew. In high school she spent more than a year without an antidepressant, all the while telling her psychiatrist she was not depressed. But both Alex and Liz had their psychiatric problems recur, in newly upsetting ways, when they reached college. What had seemed to be an easily manageable condition requiring only a small neurochemical adjustment turned out to be something that outfoxed medication. Something similar happened to a number of young people I interviewed, and, to some extent, to me, too.

In another generation, my peers and I might never have gotten any treatment, at least not until reaching a crisis point. But after being medicated for comparatively mild symptoms, many of us muddled on for years in a state of half doubt about the severity of our conditions. In one particularly interesting case, I interviewed a young man who grew up in Indiana and was medicated for mild depression at age fourteen—right around the time his older brother was diagnosed with and medicated for schizophrenia. He took the antidepressant Effexor for a couple of years, then went off it until partway through college, when his depression came back with renewed intensity, and he was again prescribed an antidepressant. But all along, regardless of how unhappy or hopeless he felt, he considered his brother the true patient. Then, upon graduating college, he experienced a psychotic depression, coupled with intrusive thoughts and obsessions about harming other people. Ultimately, he was, by his account, rescued by the antidepressant Cymbalta, the first medication that worked dramatically for him. The experience was in one sense validating, but it was also alarming since he worried that he was becoming as disturbed as his brother.

Liz found her breakdown confusing and disorienting in part because, as always, she couldn't decide either how much to expect from medication or how much to expect from herself. She kept wondering to what extent she had simply not found the right combination of drugs, and to what extent she was, as she feared, lazy, or weak, or melodramatic. My own breakdown was destabilizing for a quite different reason. Since I thought I knew just what to expect from myself and my medication, I was devastated when my cherished medication stopped working and undermined my sense of myself.

A few months after graduating from college, I accepted a job at a daily newspaper in a mid-sized Texas city on the Mexico border—one of the poorest and also one of the fastest-growing regions in the country, and utterly unlike any place I had ever lived. It was hardly the first time I'd moved to a strange city, found myself new living quarters, and begun a new job, but it was my first time doing it for an indefinite amount of time, without the reassuring end point of an internship. I had been sad to leave my boyfriend in DC, but I quickly befriended my coworkers and set myself up in a cozy apartment looking out on carefully landscaped palm trees, aloe plants, and a lovely pool. At work, I had been given the sole responsibility for reporting on an entire county, eighty miles long, where it seemed that everyone but me spoke Spanish. It was a formidable challenge, but I was determined to learn the language, the culture, and the politics of the place.

Then, about four months after I moved to Texas, I began waking up early in the morning with a jolt, and an immediate and pervasive sense of dread—of what I couldn't say. All day long, I felt at once wired and fuzzy-headed, my mind jumping from one thought to the next in a frantic, desperate race, as though each thought were a sinking ship I had to escape before being engulfed. In contrast to my high school depression, which had felt like trying to trudge through mud, I now felt frighteningly light and untethered. I was uncharacteristically fragile and weepy, as though living constantly with hypercharged PMS. A horrible, incessant churning in my stomach kept me from eating. I was unable to write. The daily deadlines terrified me, and my story ideas seemed suddenly hollow and unreal. I felt like a fraudulent ghost of my old self.

I hadn't yet found a psychiatrist in Texas, despite my mother's urgings, and was still taking the Prozac prescribed by my college health center. With no one to consult about my symptoms, I felt totally blindsided: it simply did not occur to me to attribute my breakdown either to a failure of my medication or to the extreme stress of leaving my boyfriend, my family, and my friends, relocating across the country, and beginning my first real, and really demanding, job. I didn't consider any of those factors, even in combination, cause for a breakdown; they were just things you dealt with, part of being a young, ambitious person. After I finally told my family how deeply anxious I was, my mother asked if I'd messed up my birth control pills—that, she and I both knew, could dramatically affect my mood. I told her I had. Since I'd been too anxious to remember that daily pill, it was entirely possible I hadn't been taking Prozac regularly, either. Considering the possible causes, I grew dizzy and overwhelmed, unable to keep one scenario in my head for long enough to figure out its connection to anything else.

If I had thought back to the last time I was so anxious and fragile, I might have realized that it coincided with my going off Prozac, briefly, back in college, when my hometown doctor wanted to see how I would fare without medication. But I was—as one tends to be in the midst of a psychiatric crisis—stranded in the horror of the present and steeped in dread of the immediate future. The past scarcely existed, except as a time when I had not been so frightened and desperate.

In Western culture, a certain amount of irresponsibility and "finding yourself" during the late teens and twenties is more acceptable than it was in past eras. But social mores still dictate the kind of self-exploration that's considered valid and worthwhile. In the middle- and upper-middle-class circles I grew up in, taking a gap year between high school and college to travel the world and do volunteer work is acceptable; working at Burger King is not. Graduating college and postponing law school to join Teach for America is fine; abruptly quitting your job and moving back home to live with your parents is much harder to explain. I had never wanted to dally; I'd been eager to race through to adulthood and, in particular, to take on an adult job. Since I believed a slipup or a lapse could set my career back for who knew how long, it was really saying something when, a few months after moving to South Texas, I bought a same-day, very expensive, one-way ticket to my parents' house, seriously thinking that I would have to live at home for the foreseeable future, prevented by my anxiety from ever going back.

A psychiatrist friend of my parents, who kindly agreed to see me on an emergency basis, prescribed Klonopin, the same short-term anxiety medication Elizabeth took. I was amazed and relieved when the drug immediately ratcheted down the clamor in my brain to a dull buzz, and I wanted nothing more than to curl up and hide in my childhood bedroom, surrounded by my pointe shoes and china dolls.

My parents, however, thought I should rest up for a few days, get myself together, and use the calm the Klonopin afforded to return to Texas. There, I should get a psychiatrist, adjust my antidepressants, and see if I could stick it out for a few more months at minimum, ideally staying at the job at least a year in total. If I left without warning, my mother pointed out, my bosses wouldn't be able to give me an unconditional recommendation, and I'd spend the next several years (at least) explaining why I'd left so suddenly, just five months after taking the job. Quitting would turn my private psychological turmoil into everyone's business, and even in an age when the commonly cited statistic was that one in ten adults took an antidepressant, this was not a story, she noted, that I wanted to have to keep trotting out.

My parents were right, but frankly, at the time, I was not concerned about my résumé. I still felt so diminished by the two-month-long onslaught of anxiety that, even with the short-term relief provided by the Klonopin, I couldn't conceive of having the strength or self-confidence to apply for a job anytime in the foreseeable future. In the end, my parents convinced me to return to Texas provisionally. Too weak to argue, I gave in, but with little hope I wouldn't have to fly home again in defeat.

In high school I had found therapy useless, but I now felt tenuous and vulnerable enough to think it might be grounding, even comforting. But as an outsider in a relatively isolated and insular region of Texas, I despaired of finding a therapist who would understand me or the world from which I came. Drug treatment, by contrast, had the advantage of geographical and socioeconomic neutrality. Although I couldn't imagine anything working as well as Prozac had, I imagined that a psychiatrist would only have to understand my neurotransmitters, not my neuroses, habits, quirks, and ambitions. So when the psychiatrist I found—one of only a couple in a fifty-mile radius—suggested I switch to an antidepressant called Effexor, which worked on multiple neurotransmitters and was therefore, he said, more effective for a combination of anxiety and depression, I agreed. I was in no state, frankly, to be reading scientific studies to see if he was right. Without hesitation, I tapered off the Prozac, began easing up to a therapeutic dose of Effexor and continued taking Klonopin every few hours to tamp down the anxiety when it flared.

As the months passed, my state of mind improved, but the residual anxiety and the new medications forced me to reconceptualize my view of myself in relation to my treatment. For the first time since I entered therapy as a fifteen-year-old, I saw myself as a psychiatric patient. I no longer got my prescriptions from a general practitioner or the college health center. I got them from a psychopharmacologist, and had to wait hours in a waiting area full of deeply troubled patients who babbled or stared vacantly at nothing in particular. (The office seemed to be connected to a grim-looking inpatient unit or intense day-treatment facility.) For the first time, too, I was taking a short-acting drug, Klonopin. Anxiety, my doctor had explained, spirals, and needs to be nipped in the bud. I didn't just swallow a pill unthinkingly every morning along with my allergy meds and birth control, the way I had the Prozac. Instead, I carried a little bottle of pills wherever I went, along with a bright-blue pill cutter, so I could cleanly divide a tablet when the anxiety threatened to reassert itself. The pill cutter, in particular, unnerved me, in part because, in one small swipe, it made me responsible for creating my own dose.

Effexor, too, required a new level of awareness: unlike Prozac, which is a forgiving drug, with a long-enough half-life that it rarely causes withdrawal symptoms, Effexor needs to be taken every day at the same time. If I was even a couple of hours late taking the pill, I experienced the drug's notorious "brain blips," a disorienting and hard-to-describe sensation that some people say feels like an electric shock but which to me felt more like my gray matter was being shaken around inside my skull. Prozac's side effects had been scarcely noticeable, and I could miss a dose without obvious impact. With Effexor, for the first time, I knew what it was to feel yoked to a pill.

CHAPTER 7

Side Effects

Primum non nocere. [First, do no harm.]

—MEDICAL AXIOM

I mean, I don't know if there are any statistics on this,
but how long is a person who is on psychotropic drugs supposed to live?
How long before your brain, not to mention the rest of you,
will begin to mush and deteriorate?

—ELIZABETH WURTZEL, PREFACE TO *Prozac Nation*

Elizabeth Wurtzel's memoir *Prozac Nation: Young and Depressed in America* is not, despite its title, really about the experience of being young and medicated. As the subtitle more accurately states, *Prozac Nation* is primarily about being young and depressed; Prozac doesn't even enter the picture until the very end of the book. The book does, however, open with a preface, related with the same mix of melodrama and cynicism that pervades the rest of the story, addressing certain aspects of Wurtzel's experience on medication during her early and mid-twenties. At twenty-five, she is on a cocktail: lithium and Prozac, plus a blood pressure drug and a sleeping medication. Panicking over both short- and long-term side effects, though, she concludes she "want[s] out of this life on drugs."[1]

Lithium, "the miracle salt that has stabilized my moods but is draining my body," leaves her exhausted, unable to drag herself out of bed after ten hours of sleep, and threatens to disrupt her thyroid function and make her grow fat, a fate worse than depression, she thinks. She has a tremor, and takes beta-blockers to counteract it. She worries about the long-term effects of Prozac, new on the market when she began taking it, and fantasizes about being told twenty years down the road that it has caused inoperable brain cancer. Looking at her "flushed skin" and "visible biceps" in the mirror and reflecting on how she actually *feels* on the drugs, she thinks most anyone would conclude she's on "too damn many pills."[2]

It has been nearly twenty years since Wurtzel, who later became an attorney in New York, wrote these words, and as far as I know, she has not received a diagnosis of anything so grave as inoperable brain cancer resulting from her medication use. But beyond her knowing, slightly flippant tone about this unlikely prospect are several poignant concerns that would apply, with increasing frequency, to the medicated kids in the generation following hers—the very real worry of unknown, long-term side effects, the frustration of using one drug to treat the unfortunate effects of another, and the resignation of feeling old before one's time.

Nearly all drugs, of course, psychotropic or not, prescription or over-the-counter, carry side effects that people, no matter their age, find annoying, troubling, or intolerable. Short-term side effects are one of the most common reasons for nonadherence to all manner of medications, and long-term effects are generally unknown for years following any drug's official government approval. But young people's experience of side effects from psychotropics touches on certain unique issues. Side effects can mimic symptoms, and vice versa, further complicating the already thorny task of separating drug from self from disorder. Developmentally, they often prematurely bring on health issues associated with much older people: not just the tremor Wurtzel describes, but also cognitive problems, extreme fatigue, sexual dysfunction, weight gain, heart trouble, and type 2 diabetes. In other cases, they hinder aspects of ordinary development, leaving young people lagging behind their peers—the stimulants, for example, stunt growth. What research there is shows that children and teenagers do worry about the side effects, and even about the potential for as yet unknown side effects, of psychotropics.[3] Yet, the side effects that bother someone at age ten may not be the same ones that trouble her at age fifteen, which in turn may be different from the ones that disturb her at twenty-five or thirty.

Side effects can be particularly infuriating, or simply difficult to accept, because the newer drugs that have appeared on the market in the past two decades were widely touted—not just by pharmaceutical companies, but by professional organizations and journals—as having less troublesome ancillary effects. Older antidepressants carried severe risks of food interactions and overdose. Lithium could easily reach toxic doses if a child became even slightly dehydrated running around outside. Older antipsychotics could cause lasting neurological damage—damage that, as the mental health legal scholar and author Elyn Saks poignantly notes in her memoir of schizophrenia, served as something of a scarlet letter for the mentally ill, an indication to outsiders that one was, or had been, insane.[4] Yet, with time, some of these new drugs, notably the new-generation atypical antipsychotics, have been shown to carry a high likelihood of serious side effects themselves.

It was the side effects of one such antipsychotic that turned Paul's trying experience with meds in the Florida foster-care system into an intolerable one. Ultimately, he would conclude, he'd been treated like a "guinea pig" without having had the attendant risks properly explained to him. But first, he had to discover for himself the link between his medication and the new disease he developed.

Paul, *ages fourteen to sixteen*

Paul had been taking the antipsychotic Seroquel for several years already when the most upsetting side effects emerged. From the very start, he had disliked how the drug made him feel. Drowsy and sluggish, parched and ravenous, he had stopped taking his medication while at the residential treatment center in Tampa. Once he was released on good behavior, he returned to his special behavioral school in Fort Lauderdale and reentered a therapeutic group home, the next step down from residential psychiatric treatment. This home, in an affluent suburb, seemed to Paul almost like a mansion, but a highly regimented one, including closely supervised medication dosings. A big, tough, ex-military guy handed out the pills, and unlike the nurses during Paul's final months at the Tampa facility, this staffer made sure you swallowed. *Lift up your tongue,* he'd demand. *Lemme see down your throat.*

Now that Paul was back to taking Seroquel in multiple daily doses, the hated side effects began to return. He lost the six-pack he'd had in Tampa and gained so much weight that he had rolls of fat. He was 5'4" and weighed 220 pounds. His best friend called him "Butterball," a nickname he relished—until he figured out what it meant.

Over the next few years, reports would emerge about the potential of atypical antipsychotics like Seroquel to cause obesity and diabetes. Paul's doctors seem to have been aware of at least some of these risks: they drew blood regularly and even announced on one occasion that his high blood-sugar reading put him at risk for diabetes. But Paul, as a young teenager, didn't know what diabetes was, and no one took the time to explain to him what it meant or to suggest he modify his diet or get more exercise.

Certainly, the prospect of switching to a medication with fewer side effects was not discussed (some atypicals carry a lower risk of metabolic effects, while mood stabilizers, such as the Tegretol Paul had previously been on, are also used in the treatment of bipolar disorder and generally have less pernicious side effects).[5] Paul did play on the basketball team at school, which in theory offered some exercise, but he found it easy to get out of both practice and games. One day, when Paul was in eighth grade, an announcement went out over the school loudspeakers for the basketball players to report to the locker room for a game. Paul was feeling particularly unmotivated, so he decided to play sick, the old standby of recalcitrant kids everywhere. In fact, he felt fine, well enough that he'd gulped down two big Sunny Delight orange juice containers and three honey buns at the school cafeteria that morning. When he feigned sickness, he got himself dispatched to the school nurse.

At the nurse's office, Paul complained of feeling drowsy and woozy.

The nurse, who would have known he took psychotropic medications, took his blood pressure and made a face indicating disbelief. Then she called in Paul's school therapist, whom he saw twice a week for counseling, and the two conferred in the back room in hushed voices. The therapist returned and asked kindly, "Paul, are you okay?" Still trying to look as ill as possible to get out of the basketball game, Paul didn't say anything, so the therapist persisted. "Paul, I need you to be one hundred percent honest with me. Are you on drugs?" "No, I'm not on drugs," Paul said, a little petulantly. By drugs, of course, they meant illegal drugs, since they knew he took Seroquel. The therapist kept pressing. "Are you *sure* you're not on drugs?" When Paul insisted he wasn't, the nurse and therapist exchanged worried looks, and the nurse said she was going to call 911.

An ambulance came, and the paramedics loaded him onto a stretcher, even though Paul protested that he really had to pee. They insisted there was no time to waste, and gave him a bucket to relieve himself in on the way. Lying in the ambulance, staring at the cords hanging from the ceiling, Paul considered his situation. *Shit*, he thought, *how am I going to get out of this? There is* NOTHING WRONG WITH ME. Actually getting to go to the hospital because he'd faked sick was half thrilling and half galling. He was impressed with himself for taking the scheme this far, but he also wasn't looking forward to being chewed out by his therapist, his foster-care caseworker, his basketball coach, and everyone else for creating such an unnecessary scene.

At the hospital, an assistant took his blood, and a team of doctors came in and questioned him. One of them said, "I can't believe you are talking to me right now. You should be in a coma." Paul was nonplussed. Instead, he considered his grumbling stomach. "I'm hungry," he said. "Can I have something to eat?" Everyone looked at him in horror. "Absolutely not," the doctor said. "You're not eating anything until your blood sugar goes down *dramatically*. You're a diabetic." They gave him some ice chips to suck on and waited for his blood sugar to return to an acceptable range. It took more than twelve hours, and it was past midnight before Paul got anything to eat.

Meanwhile, the doctors explained the problem: Paul had type 2 diabetes. Untreated, it had caused a potentially fatal reaction. That scared him. Was being a diabetic like having HIV? Did it mean he was going to die? Would he ever be able to get married and have kids? The hospital staffers did their best to reassure him. Diabetes was absolutely treatable, they said—Paul would simply have to learn how to give himself insulin injections to make up for what his body couldn't produce on its own. To Paul, that sounded worse than HIV, worse than anything he could imagine. Whenever he had been hospitalized or institutionalized for psychiatric problems, the use of a needle meant the patient was acting up and needed to be sedated. A needle represented the ultimate capitulation. Paul was not one to capitulate.

He was also not particularly stoic about the pain. The first time he had to give himself a shot, he nearly passed out—it *hurt*. He couldn't do this three times a day for the rest of his life. From then on, every time he had to prick himself to check his blood sugar or inject himself with insulin, he felt a wave of sadness and defeat come over him. So far, he'd been very good at manipulating his circumstances to suit his purposes, but diabetes seemed one thing he couldn't wiggle out of. His alleged behavior problems were finally under control, and at the residential psychiatric center at least he'd been able to spit out the Seroquel. But failure to inject himself, everyone told him, would put his life in danger.

At some point, Paul's psychiatrist explained that his diabetes probably resulted from taking Seroquel. Paul wondered why doctors would prescribe him a drug that caused another illness, but he figured at first that they knew what they were doing. As he got a little older, he also made a connection between the diabetes and other side effects of Seroquel that he disliked so much—the dry mouth, the cravings, the woozy, dizzy feeling. Once when he had either forgotten to take his Seroquel the night before or his foster parents had forgotten to give it to him, he awoke without a dry mouth, and it occurred to him that maybe he could avoid that feeling if he didn't take the pills. So he went a week without taking them. He felt better, and saw that his blood sugar readings were more level. Then, the morning after he'd gone back to taking the drug, he awoke with a dry, fat-feeling tongue and abnormal blood sugar again. Finally, he understood the connection—and realized that maybe the diabetes was reversible if he stopped taking his medication. This was a revelation. As he'd understood it, he'd have to deal with the condition for the rest of his life.

By the time Paul figured this out, he had moved away from the group home and was living in a different therapeutic foster-care placement, one chosen for him because the father was a nurse and could monitor his condition. Both parents watched like hawks while Paul took his insulin and his Seroquel, nagged him to go out and get some exercise to lose weight and control his blood sugar, and monitored his whereabouts and his grades. Later, he would see the discipline they imposed as beneficial, but for the moment he chafed at being stuck adhering to two different medical treatments he intensely disliked, one of which—the Seroquel—seemed to be maddeningly and needlessly causing the other.

In time, with his diabetes under control, Paul was transferred to a more relaxed foster home where, now aged sixteen or so, he was put in charge of his own medication. He stopped taking Seroquel altogether, and noticed himself shedding weight. Eventually, his blood sugar problems disappeared, and his doctor told him he no longer needed insulin. He felt vindicated.

Paul has been vindicated many times since, as more and more evidence has emerged showing that atypical antipsychotics drastically increase the risk of metabolic symptoms, such as obesity and diabetes, in children and teenagers. In the past decade, a growing number of studies have found an elevated risk of these conditions in adults, and in 2003 the FDA required drug companies to print diabetes warnings on drug labels.[6] Since then, studies have shown that children who take atypical antipsychotics are even more vulnerable to rapid weight gain and high blood sugar than adults.[7] (More recently, studies have examined whether the weight gain from the atypicals might be helpful in treating anorexia, by improving mood and, yes, inducing weight gain.)

During the past few years, evidence has also mounted indicating that several major pharmaceutical companies knowingly failed to disclose these risks and that some of the most prominent academic psychiatrists promoting drug use in children took large sums as speakers or consultants for pharmaceutical companies. Thousands of patient lawsuits proliferated, and several major drug manufacturers also ended up reaching settlements with the government on charges they illegally marketed the drugs without FDA approval for a given condition or population, including for use in children.[8] In 2010 AstraZeneca, the maker of Seroquel, joined the list, accepting a fine of $520 million in response to government charges that it promoted the drug off-label, including to children, and paid kickbacks to doctors.[9] This story of influence peddling has been well chronicled elsewhere, notably in the *New York Times*'s relentless coverage, in former *Times* reporter Melody Petersen's book on the pharmaceutical industry, *Our Daily Meds*, and in psychiatrist and blogger Daniel Carlat's insider's look at drug company influence, *Unhinged: The Trouble with Psychiatry.*

As alarming as Paul's experience with Seroquel was, at least he could seemingly link his dangerous side effects to his medication—there was a clear relationship between taking Seroquel, his blood sugar readings, and how he felt physically. Caleb experienced similar side effects from the antipsychotic Zyprexa: thirty pounds of rapid weight gain; six years later he ruefully showed me the shiny white stretch marks across his hips. But Caleb considered Zyprexa a not-unreasonable attempt to reign in his wild manias and excruciating mixed states. Paul, in contrast, never considered his moods a problem, at least not a problem that could be remedied with drugs. Instead, he pinned his hopes for happiness on being adopted, probably a far-fetched dream, given his serious behavior problems. In retrospect, Paul considered Seroquel a risky, even dangerous, choice on the part of the people who were supposed to be looking out for him.

The metabolic side effects associated with the new antipsychotics are by now well established, though the information was sparser when today's young adults began taking these medications as children or teens. The sexual side effects of SSRI antidepressants, however, have been well known and widely reported in both scientific literature and the mainstream media since the early 1990s. But when it came to children and adolescents, and even young adults, they simply weren't discussed. Between 1991 and 2002, the FDA's adverse event reporting system received just eight reports of SSRI-induced sexual dysfunction in adolescents. A comprehensive review of the literature conducted in 2004 found just one clinical trial that reported erectile dysfunction in a teenager; most clinical guidelines and reviews of SSRIs didn't mention sexual side effects at all.[10]

That is pretty shocking since, as the author of the study cited above noted, anywhere from 30 to 40 percent of adults experience some kind of SSRI-induced problems with libido, arousal, or orgasm.[11] Perhaps clinicians and researchers just didn't think to ask—adults are known to underreport sexual side effects of SSRIs unless specifically asked, and teens are likely to be even more secretive. A 2001 article in the *Journal of Child and Adolescent Psychopharmacology* dryly concluded that "most teens would rather become non-compliant [taking the drugs] than start a discussion about the effect of the medication on their sexual experience."[12] If true, that may be because they suspected they wouldn't be taken seriously, and might even be judged harshly. American culture tends to regard child and even teenage sexual behavior more as a menace than as a natural part of life. Teen pregnancy rates had spiked in the late 1980s, and although rates subsequently decreased to a twenty-year low by the end of the 1990s, the subject of sex among teenagers was a significant cultural concern and political preoccupation, as reflected by an outpouring of government funds for abstinence-only sex education and efforts to limit children's exposure to sexually explicit content on television.[13]

The experts also have little sense of the long-term effects of drugs on sexual functioning into adulthood, except that animal studies of young rats given Prozac show decreased sexual behavior as adults.[14] The SSRIs are the psychotropics most likely to cause sexual side effects, though certain mood stabilizers can also have those effects. Despite the lack of formal studies involving young people, anecdotal evidence suggests that drugs causing decreased libido and sexual functioning do sometimes pose a real problem, psychologically and socially, both for teenagers who are in the process of developing a sexual identity and for young adults testing out long-term intimate relationships.

For Elizabeth, antidepressants had affected her sex drive from the time she first started taking them, in ninth grade. Compared to her friends, it seemed she just wasn't as interested in sex, or as inclined to pursue sexual relationships. In twelfth grade, when her first boyfriend was pressuring her to have sex, she wasn't holding out for the usual reasons; she just didn't have any desire to do it. She switched from one SSRI to another in hopes of increasing her libido, but when she did have sex with her boyfriend, it was terribly painful. She tried to detach mentally, but found herself gritting her teeth and just hoping it would be over as soon as possible. After that first relationship in high school, she did hook up with other people, but didn't have intercourse again until she was twenty-five. Whenever a relationship seemed promising, she would broach the possibility of little or no sex (few of the guys were enthusiastic at the prospect). Regardless of what they agreed to, she felt constantly pressured, and the pressure exacerbated her anxiety. That, in turn, contributed to a condition in which she tensed up muscles in her vagina, which made contact painful. Liz put the overall impact this way:

> I am not sure I can [over]state the extent to which it impacted things. I didn't grow up with a normal sex drive, and that was obviously due to a combination of factors, but being on and off antidepressants whose impact I really couldn't understand back when I didn't have any real understanding of my sex drive or sex in relationships to begin with means I basically went through adolescence without experiencing anything in that realm in a "normal" way.

I also discovered a poignant post on an Internet forum from a young woman that read: "How to begin? I might as well get to the point. I have lost all sensation in my vagina. Sex doesn't feel like much of anything to me." The young woman had been taking either Celexa or Lexapro since age fifteen, when she was diagnosed with bipolar disorder. She also took Depakote, a mood stabilizer that can affect sex drive and functioning. "I never even realized that the two things could be related until recently. I figured it was just something wrong with me," she wrote, adding that she would be switching from Celexa to Wellbutrin, a drug known for having less impact on sex drive. She concluded by saying she was excited and anxious: "Has anyone else been through this? What can I expect during the transition? Is there hope for me?" Older people who take medication for comparatively mild troubles and experience sexual side effects can remember what they were like before the drugs, assess the change, and make a cost-benefit analysis: if sexual problems aren't worth the benefits of the drugs, ditch the meds. (In fact, sexual problems are thought to be a major reason that a high percentage of adults receiving SSRIs don't refill their initial prescriptions.) The calculus changes, however, when one begins taking medication during a time of developing sexuality. There is the possibility, first of all, that the sexual symptoms are actually signs of the disorder itself—depression can cause decreased libido, anxiety can contribute to problems with arousal and orgasm, and, on the other side of the equation, mania is often characterized by hypersexuality. Then there's the question of what's "normal" in terms of sex drive, arousal, and orgasm. With the typical teenage or college-aged boy, who may well be oversexed, it might not be such a bad thing for a female partner if his libido is somewhat reduced or his orgasm delayed a little (indeed, SSRIs are prescribed off-label to treat premature ejaculation). One guy I interviewed who took SSRIs for anxiety while attending high school in New Jersey was sure they decreased arousal and diminished orgasm—but since his girlfriend wanted to have sex multiple times in succession, he regarded his apparent drug-induced limitations with a grain of salt.

Of course, not being able to achieve and maintain an erection is embarrassing and emasculating for men of all ages—witness the blockbuster success of Viagra. Young guys, who are supposed to be the picture of virility and whose peers place a huge value on sex, are likely to be even more disturbed by these problems. Another young man I interviewed had had sex before he began taking antidepressants, but thought they had profoundly affected how he viewed sex, as well as his friendships and romantic relationships. On various antidepressants, he had trouble staying aroused and orgasming; especially in college, the trouble made him wary of getting into any potential sexual situation.

He drank to combat his performance anxiety, which probably only made his performance worse, he later acknowledged. Not only was he ashamed in his sexual encounters, but his problems made him feel estranged from his male friends. "I mean, sure, I could make stuff up, or act like everything was awesome (I'm sure some guys who aren't even on meds do that), but that would feel hollow and make me feel fake and worse than if I just stayed quiet," he said. Throughout, he wondered how much his problems could be attributed to meds, versus some unknown psychological hang-up, and he wondered, too, how he could ever have a meaningful and intimate romantic relationship without satisfying sex.

Both young men and women also face the question of whether to disclose to their partner the source of the problems. Not everyone wants to admit to taking psychiatric medication, especially to a one-time hookup. Even admitting sexual side effects to a more serious, long-term partner who knows about one's treatment—and not all of them do—isn't necessarily a get-out-of-jail-free card. It can provoke unwelcome and unsolicited opinions about one's treatment, or just more subtle pressure, as was the case for Liz.

Many people said they didn't experience sexual problems attributable to meds, but when I inquired about the subject, they admitted that never having had sex before going on medication, and never having spent significant time off medication, they had no basis for comparison. When I asked Claire about this in her new house in Seattle, where she lives with her husband, she laughed a little and said none of that stuff had ever been a problem for her. Her husband interjected to say that because she had been taking the drugs since she was eleven, she wouldn't really know. Claire conceded he had a point.

Claire, ages eleven to twenty-five
OHIO AND CALIFORNIA / 1991–2005

One thing Claire knew to be a problem, long before she went on medication, was her sleeping patterns. As she recounted in *Claire's Story*, her video about childhood and teen depression, she had slept poorly from infancy, and the first sign of her depression, in fact, was persistent insomnia. Even after going on antidepressants, she had trouble sleeping and was often exhausted during the day—on occasion falling asleep in class, to her classmates' amusement. In college, her friends joked that if they weren't talking directly to her, she'd doze off. To some extent, sleepiness was just a family trait. Some families get together for meals and then watch football; after eating, hers would conk out in the living room. But, since her sleeping problems had worsened with the appearance of her depression, and since they persisted for years after she began taking medication, she and her parents concluded that this was an untreated symptom of her disorder.

There was something to this conclusion. In fact, doctors have long known that people with depression are prone to disturbed sleep patterns, and studies have shown that antidepressants, even when they treat other symptoms of the disorder, sometimes fail to fix sleep troubles such as evening or early-morning insomnia, or intermittent nighttime awakenings. This failure to resolve the underlying problems, even when other depressive symptoms remit, may, in turn, increase the risk of relapse and perhaps even of suicidality. Some antidepressants, moreover, actually appear to worsen sleep beyond any preexisting depression-related disturbances.[15]

A couple of years after graduating college, Claire switched from SSRIs, which she had been alternating between almost constantly since age eleven, to Cymbalta, which works on the neurotransmitter norepinephrine as well as serotonin. She noticed a significant change in her sleep patterns. For the first time since she could remember, she was able to get up in the morning—voluntarily—before 9 a.m. Naps were optional, not necessary. It began to seem as if she'd reversed cause and effect. Rather than failing to treat the exhaustion that came along with her depression, perhaps her previous antidepressants had made her sleepier. This was a curious possibility to consider, that something that had for years not only dictated her daily routine but in some ways defined her was an incidental effect of the drug. For years, especially during the time she spoke publicly about her experience with depression, she hadn't minded defining herself as a kid with depression and considered her need for sleep simply an example of how she could treat—but not cure—such a condition.

By the time she went on Cymbalta, quite a lot had changed. She had tempered the activist persona she'd adopted as a teenager: blurting out that she had depression and was on meds was, she joked in retrospect, no longer the first thing she announced on meeting someone. She also wondered whether, now that she was in her mid-twenties, her body clock had reset itself and she no longer needed as much rest. Finally, her symptoms were beginning to shift around this time. Her last major depressive breakdown had occurred a couple of years earlier, right after graduating from college. Although she had suffered what she called "anxiety storms" since early childhood, she now had more frequent and longer-lasting episodes characterized less by fatigue and more by hyperactivity and jitteriness: with her pressured speech, she seemed to others almost manic, but she knew she was just overcompensating for the terror by talking a mile a minute. Doctors prescribed Klonopin to calm her, but that made her immediately—and obviously—very sleepy. As a teacher, she had to be able to get up in the morning and command a room of unruly middle schoolers. Klonopin was out.

An intense need for sleep and daytime drowsiness have also been problems for me at least since I began taking antidepressants more than a decade ago. For a long time I maintained that I was just one of those people who needed lots of sleep, and lectured friends who slept less, saying they didn't know how impaired they were. But my lingering daytime tiredness has me wondering if I was wrong about myself—if turning into someone who on some fundamental level needed lots of sleep was a side effect of my medication. Drowsiness is a potential side effect of practically every psychotropic drug, except the stimulants. Wellbutrin, the antidepressant I've taken for five years, is supposedly "activating," but most of the time I have also been taking an SSRI antidepressant to help temper my anxiety, and those might well make me sleepy. Or maybe, as Claire had surmised about her own situation before trying Cymbalta, my underlying depression is mostly treated by the meds, but the disrupted sleep remains.

Doctors have not been very sympathetic. My primary care physicians keep testing for thyroid problems, vitamin deficiencies, and the like. My psychiatrists say, "Well, maybe you're just someone who needs a lot of sleep." We've broached the topic of my taking some sort of stimulant, like Provigil, to counteract the effects of the other meds; I know other people who do this. But the idea of adding a drug to treat the side effects of another drug vaguely disturbs me, as it does many people.

In fact, clinical guidelines often mention this kind of augmentation to deal with the common side effects of psychotropics—Ritalin to counteract decreased libido and weight gain, Viagra for problems with sexual arousal, Wellbutrin for both sexual problems and drowsiness. Each, of course, carries its own potential side effects, and multiple drugs complicate the task of assessing one's progress. They also have the effect of making you feel *old*, as Elizabeth Wurtzel noted in *Prozac Nation*. It's dismaying to have a long line of pill bottles in the medicine cabinet, or, perhaps worse, larger and larger pill organizers to help you keep track of when you need to take what.

Of course, many of the side effects themselves carry connotations of premature aging: Type 2 diabetes from the atypical antipsychotics; impotence and loss of libido and sexual functioning from SSRIs and mood stabilizers; memory problems and other cognitive deficits from antianxiety meds like Klonopin and Xanax; difficulty remembering words from certain mood stabilizers; and mental fogginess and tremors from various drugs. Children probably aren't aware of this perverse irony, that the drugs meant to help them enjoy a long and full life carry with them whispers of old age, but teens and young adults are more conscious of it. One man I interviewed who had tried newer antidepressants without effect described the peculiar sensation of ferrying home Metamucil from the drugstore in order to treat the constipation caused by his tricyclic antidepressant. All of a sudden he felt terribly old.

Then again, some aspects of mental illness rob you of your youth, or, alternatively, leave you behind while your peers surge ahead. Depression steals one's enthusiasm, libido, vivaciousness. Anxiety takes away the feeling of youthful invulnerability. Going from the highs of mania and to the lows of depression provides a particularly dramatic and brutal lesson in the repercussions of impulsiveness and risk-taking. ADHD, which experts increasingly view as a delay in brain development, often leaves children and especially teens lagging while their peers progress.

Medications for ADHD, though, can cause side effects that make people feel either older or younger. The shorter-acting ones, for example, wear off and can cause irritable meltdowns that resemble toddlers' temper tantrums. On the other hand, they are also known to raise heart rate and blood pressure in both children and adults, and have been associated in very rare cases with sudden deaths in both populations, although nearly half of the child deaths on record had existing cardiac structural abnormalities.[16] The drugs' ability to reduce impulsiveness can make many kids feel less carefree and more inhibited. One young man from Arizona who began taking stimulants and antidepressants in second grade for ADHD blamed the inhibiting effects of the drugs for making it impossible for him to chat up girls in high school.

Although comparatively short-acting and sometimes taken less often as kids mature and develop coping skills, stimulants may have side effects that have a lasting impact on how young people view themselves. One is their potential to stunt growth. Certainly, smaller kids often get teased or bullied in school. Yet, the detrimental effects can continue into adulthood: as numerous studies have demonstrated, height correlates with higher pay, better jobs, and romantic success, especially for men. Another potential legacy is the creation of a problematic relationship to food: once sold as diet drugs, stimulants curb appetite. One young woman described to me with frustration how, while her peers learned to control their food urges, stimulants made it so she never had to. She ate so little on the drugs that by the time they wore off each day in the afternoon or evening, she could binge without gaining weight. After high school, she took a year off to travel and went off her medications. Unused to eating in moderation, she rapidly gained a lot of weight, which she only lost through crash dieting. It took years before she learned to recalibrate her eating habits. She knew plenty of other girls her age with "food issues," but most of them had at least learned a measure of self-control that, thanks to her years on stimulants, she seemed to lack.

Some people take comfort in blaming medications for one ailment or another; it absolves them of responsibility. This is particularly easy to do in retrospect, for drugs one no longer takes, as one feels no allegiance to them. Those of us who have taken meds long term, however, tend to be sensitive about accusations that we are failing to exercise a sufficient "mind over matter" approach. We want to believe that the drugs enable us to be our true and full selves. Yet, sexuality, body image, and the energy for sociability are all important to the sense of self that develops in adolescence and young adulthood. To have any of these compromised serves as an unpleasant reminder that we're less empowered than we think.

CHAPTER 8

Complicating Factors

It isn't often that headlines from trade publications stick with me, but I was struck by this one from *Psychiatric Times*, a widely read newsletter for psychiatrists: "The Meaning of Life in a 15-Minute Med Check." The hyperbole of the claim highlights the larger question: how can a doctor address the meaning of *anything*, let alone of life, in so short and regimented a span of time?

The article's author, a psychiatrist at the Medical College of Wisconsin who studies cultural psychiatry and the ethics of care, provides a novel answer: near the beginning of appointments, he has taken to asking his patients what gives meaning to their lives. This not only helps patients feel invested in their own care but also helps him direct his treatment decisions toward improving their quality of life. He notes that this approach may be especially effective with teenagers, who are just beginning to ponder what gives their lives meaning. His question, although tinged with positivity, provides a way of getting at deeply troubling issues that the more typical focus on narrowly defined symptoms and physiological side effects does not.[1]

Because a short "medication management" session cannot comprehensively deal with the more complicated issues of adolescence and early adulthood, young patients must either rely on their medication and their own devices, or supplement their fifteen-minute psychiatric consultations with talk therapy, if they can afford to do so. I was struck by how many young people I interviewed reported feeling slighted, misunderstood, or just alienated by their prescribing doctors and craved a closer relationship, especially as children but also as they entered adulthood. On the other hand, plenty of my peers are happy to get their prescriptions and run; in fact, several said they'd like to eliminate the doctor as middleman altogether. As Caleb put it, "The only thing stopping me from writing my own prescriptions is the law. That signature at the bottom of the scrip is worth $125 a visit." I have felt this way myself in the past, especially when I was stable, when my meds were working, and my relationship with my prescribing doctor perfunctory.

Yet, regardless of how patients feel about their doctors' limited roles, the problem with this approach to psychiatric treatment is that medication, life experiences, and other health issues often overlap in confusing ways. A number of complicating factors loom especially large in adolescence and young adulthood: coming to terms with sexuality and sexual orientation, experimenting with alcohol and drugs, and certain health concerns, such as becoming pregnant for the first time. Many of these issues are complicated or exacerbated by taking meds, even as the issues themselves complicate or exacerbate the challenges of monitoring and adhering to medications. With parents who grew up in an era far less dominated by psychiatric medication and doctors who are often either too busy or out of touch to provide helpful guidance, young patients find themselves struggling to understand how their substance use, health, and sexuality affect and are affected by their medications.

Alex, ages eighteen to twenty-two

BROOKLYN AND LONG ISLAND, NEW YORK / 2006–2010

Alex's first conscious consideration of his sexual orientation came when he was ten years old, during a breakdown that resulted in a diagnosis of obsessive-compulsive disorder and a prescription for an SSRI. His initial obsession—fearing he was adopted—subsided after a couple of weeks only to give way to what for him was an equally disturbing thought: the worry that he was gay. The concern, by all appearances, was purely abstract. Alex wasn't aware of feeling attracted to other boys and hadn't engaged in any same-sex sexual behavior. He couldn't say why the thought was so upsetting, except that, like his earlier adoption worries, it seemed to have appeared out of nowhere and now seemed lodged in his brain, bearing down on him with painful intensity.

Alex didn't know it at the time, but in fact, an obsessive worry about being gay is a not-uncommon preoccupation for teens and young adults suffering from OCD, even if they know they are straight. Although the psychiatric profession characterized homosexuality as a disorder until 1973 and some religious groups still advocate "conversion" therapy, mainstream practice by the time of Alex's homosexuality worries in the late 1990s would likely have based treatment decisions on whether a clinician judged the worry to be based on justified concerns, about stigma, for example, or whether the patient was beset by irrational fears suggesting OCD. The former called for counseling or talk therapy to explore the source of the conflicts and make peace with his sexual orientation, whatever it might be; the latter, as symptoms of OCD, would be better treated with medication or short-term cognitive-behavioral therapy. In this case, ten-year-old Alex's worries seemed to have no logical basis—he couldn't explain *why* he was so worried. Years later, he couldn't recall either his therapist or his psychiatrist making much of the concerns. When his fears subsided, he and his mother assumed that Luvox had successfully dealt with the issue.

But a few years later, Alex, still taking Luvox, began to think differently about the prospect of being gay. In seventh grade he had a big crush on an older girl, but the next year he became aware of being much more attracted to other boys. He brushed off his interest in his male classmates as envy: so many of them were athletic and buff, and he had never been physically fit. In contrast to his ever-present worry at age ten over being gay, he was now able to put the thought out of his head. Although he wasn't afraid of being teased, and knew his mother accepted gay people, homosexuality would nonetheless have involved some mental gymnastics, not least because ever since kindergarten he had been taught by his Catholic schoolteachers that homosexuality was a sin (later, he would formulate his own opinions, based on his reading of theology).

At the beginning of high school, Alex developed a lasting interest in a boy, let's call him Tom, who had initially struck Alex as a bully but who ended up impressing and surprising Alex with his intelligence and flashes of kindness. Alex later recognized that he'd had a crush on the kid, but at the time he only half admitted it to himself—and certainly didn't mention it to Tom or anyone else. Meanwhile, his obsessions remained in check, and in tenth grade, he tapered off his medication.

Shortly after graduating from high school, however, Alex sank into an acute depression. Clashing with his stepfather and estranged from his formerly doting mother, he felt very much in need of support and began to panic about never seeing Tom again. Although they had never been close, Alex for some reason began to consider Tom as someone he could turn to for support. He sent the boy an e-mail, making sure to keep the tone light and cheery. Over the summer, Alex sent an e-mail every two or three weeks, and received short, neutral responses. He spent hours planning the messages, terrified of scaring Tom away by appearing too desperate or clingy. Even though there was nothing in the e-mails to suggest Alex had any romantic or sexual interest in the boy, it was clear that Tom was becoming more and more disturbed by Alex's behavior. And yet, Alex couldn't stop thinking about the boy, or bring himself to break off the correspondence. Then, one day, Alex called his former classmate on the phone. Tom threatened violence if Alex didn't stop. Despite his depressed, clouded state, Alex could see the rejection was final.

Even years later, Alex refused to disclose the details of this last phone call, except to say that it precipitated another severe depressive episode, including a day spent virtually catatonic in bed. When Alex emerged from this paralysis, he returned to obsessing over his interactions with Tom with renewed fervor. The two of them had always gotten along in high school, so why did the kid not want to be friends now? Did Alex have some terrible personal deficiency he was unaware of? Would the kid have acted differently if Alex had been able to explain he was in the midst of a breakdown with no one else to turn to?

From then on, Alex continued to ruminate about the falling-out, his worries intensifying along with his depression. Back in high school, he had taken pleasure in thinking about Tom. Now these thoughts monopolized him, tore at his brain, and he wished desperately to be rid of them. Alex told both his psychiatrist and therapist about these obsessions, which seemed to him clearly pathological. What the psychiatrist made of them was unclear since he tended to talk little, even deferring to Alex about adjustments to his medications. The therapist had a very different reaction. He thought Alex was denying his homosexuality and suggested repeatedly that Alex would be less tormented if he were to pursue a healthy sexual relationship with another man—someone who, unlike his former classmate, was actually interested in him.

Alex conceded that he was attracted to men, but bristled at the suggestion that the only way to resolve his obsession was to embrace homosexuality. A devout Catholic who studied religious philosophy, he was firmly opposed to such a relationship, as the Catholic Church holds that sex between men is immoral since it cannot lead to procreation. Also, Alex didn't think pursuing a relationship with another guy while constantly obsessing about Tom would be a wise strategy. What Alex didn't tell his therapist, but what he would later recognize as an important factor in his reasoning, was that the prospect of putting himself out there scared him. To comfort himself and also, he realized later, to preclude the possibility of being attractive to others, Alex began overeating. Perhaps the therapist sensed this and thought a relationship would help Alex overcome his fears, but Alex was not having any of it. He told the therapist he would not be coming back.

The mental health profession has long had a fraught relationship with homosexuality, not to mention other forms of "nontraditional" sexual behavior and gender identity. Freud in fact promulgated a fairly tolerant view of homosexuality for his time, emphasizing that it was not a pathology, but a sign of immature psychosexual development because it involved deriving pleasure from other sex acts besides penile-vaginal intercourse.[2] Later psychoanalysts, especially in the United States, interpreted homosexual attraction as a fear of heterosexuality resulting from a distant father and overprotective mother. Erik Erikson, the father of developmental psychology, saw homosexuality as a rejection of parental and societal values after a young person had failed to assume a positive, acceptable identity.[3] In the early 1970s, the gay rights movement succeeded in lobbying the American Psychiatric

Association to remove homosexuality from the *Diagnostic and Statistical Manual of Mental Disorders*, although for several years afterward the *DSM* listed as a disorder conflicted ideas about homosexuality. The major American mental health professional organizations formally renounced the notion of same-sex attraction as pathological,[4] but since then they have varied in their approach to treating gay patients. The American Psychological Association publishes guidelines for treating LGBT (lesbian, gay, bisexual, and transgender) patients, but the organizations composed of doctors who actually prescribe the meds have had less to say on the matter in recent decades. Their silence may reflect psychiatry's uncomfortable legacy with homosexuality, but probably has more to do with the influence of biological psychiatry, which concerns itself with the diagnosis and treatment of disorders: if same-sex attractions aren't disorders, they aren't relevant to modern psychiatric practice. The psychopharmaceutical revolution of the 1980s and 1990s furthered this view. As the psychiatrist Jonathan Metzl points out in *Prozac on the Couch*, his study of gender and psychopharmaceuticals, one of the advantages of such drugs is their very neutrality—the fact that they would, in theory, "work largely the same in men and women, white and brown, gay and straight."[5]

Alex's case, involving obsessive worries about being gay that initially responded to meds, followed by same-sex urges and finally a disturbing obsession with another boy, offers a particularly telling example of the ways that disorders, medications, and psychosocial factors intersect in complicated ways. Indeed, clinicians and academics who argue for integrated therapy and medication treatment can rightly point to the larger issue of developing sexuality as yet another area where treating young people requires extra nuance and sensitivity. Miriam Rosenberg, a psychiatrist working outside Boston who has several decades of experience treating young LGBT patients, has argued that psychiatrists who fail to inquire about sexual orientation risk treating patients for symptoms that actually stem from concerns about their sexual or gender orientation. And, she says, given psychiatry's history with homosexuality, kids have good reason to be less than forthcoming. "Many adolescents are aware that only a few years ago they could have been involuntarily hospitalized and subjected to hormone and shock treatment solely on the basis of being gay," she wrote in a 2003 article in the *Journal of the American Academy of Child and Adolescent Psychiatry*. Rosenberg believes that the stigma, shame, and isolation associated with growing up gay, lesbian, bisexual, or transgender often creates symptoms of anxiety, depression, post-traumatic stress (from severe bullying), and even psychosis. In those cases, medication can be enormously helpful, but, she argues, it's also important for the doctor to create a warm and welcoming space where teens feel comfortable discussing their sexuality.[6]

For the past two decades, same-sex-attracted teens have often been treated with meds while their concerns about coming out, stigma, and bullying went either unaddressed, or were addressed in venues apart from their psychiatric treatment, such as gay-straight alliances in schools, Internet chat rooms, after-school hangouts, and counseling programs. Meanwhile, to further confuse things, they received strong messages about mental health that emphasized social influences. In the 1980s and 1990s, research into the experience of gay adolescents boomed, presenting an unrelenting picture of these teens as disproportionately afflicted with mental illness resulting from stigma, including attempting suicide at disproportionately high rates. More recently, some researchers, notably Ritch Savin-Williams of Cornell, in his 2005 book *The New Gay Teenager*, have argued that these heavily publicized statistics relied on samples of kids who were gay but also had other troubles, which created a skewed portrait of "suffering suicidal" teens.[7]

For kids who are struggling with their sexuality, the question, then, becomes this: How much can they expect from medication? If stigma, homophobia, and discrimination caused or sparked their psychiatric problems, they might well view drugs as a temporary solution—maybe welcome, maybe not—until they can transition to a more accepting environment. Or, they may conclude that preexisting psychiatric problems exacerbated the difficulties of belonging to a sexual minority. Medications, if they work, can ease the bumps inherent in any stressful situation, but they provide no guarantee of long-term stability and peace of mind.

• • •

Gay kids are hardly the only ones reluctant to talk about sex with a doctor. My peers and I grew up in a casual hookup culture where having "friends with benefits" and bootie calls by late-night text message were common practice. Many of us, especially during college, don't like the fact that there seems to be no middle ground between exclusive, long-term relationships and random hookups, but participate because that's simply how things are. Older generations, however, are habitually alarmed by what the younger ones do with regard to sex, and many clinicians middle-aged and older are long married and have forgotten what they themselves did in their youth. There is a danger that they may interpret young, single people's frequent, and frequently drunken, hookups as pathological hypersexuality, or as hallmark symptoms of mania and hypomania, or an attempt to assuage depression and anxiety. By eliminating the need to discuss sexuality at length—at least beyond the brief discussions of sexual dysfunction caused by some drugs—medication-only treatment may cause the clinician to miss some indications of trouble, but it can also protect today's young adults from feared disapproval and misdiagnosis.

Another factor that can be complicated by the generation gap between patients and medical professionals is substance use or abuse. For decades, researchers have recognized that alcohol and drug use tends to peak in the late teens, then declines as young people move into the workforce, marry, have children, and generally settle down. The percentage of young people engaging in heavy drinking has increased over the past two to three decades, and has been widely chronicled in the media. Federal statistics from 2009 show that in a given month, 42 percent of those eighteen to twenty-five reported binge drinking (defined as consuming five or more drinks in one sitting) at least once, compared to 28 percent in 1988. Among those twenty-six to thirty-four, 36 percent binge drank, compared to 20 percent in 1988. Rates among college students are even higher, although the use of illegal drugs is higher among nonstudents. Parents and educators are forever wringing their hands over heavy alcohol consumption—and several high-profile alcohol-poisoning deaths on college campuses have arguably given them good reason to do so—but the fact is that this mode of drinking is widespread through one's early thirties.[8]

Clinicians treating young people with psychotropics, however, have good reason to suspect that heavy drinking or drug use may be problematic, since comorbid substance abuse is more common for psychiatric patients than the general population.[9] It's often assumed that people with substance abuse issues are merely self-medicating for untreated psychological troubles, but in fact some studies point to the contrary. One large epidemiological survey that controlled for the comorbidity of substance use disorders found that adults with anxiety disorders who took psychiatric meds were significantly *more* likely to self-medicate with drugs or alcohol than those who didn't undergo treatment. They also scored lower on quality-of-life indicators and had a more impaired overall level of functioning.[10] These patients appeared, in other words, to be both medicating and self-medicating. The few studies specifically devoted to young people taking psychiatric meds suggest that these people are more likely to binge drink, smoke cigarettes, and take illegal drugs than their nonmedicated peers.

There simply isn't enough data, however, to explain why this would be the case—and whether it is pathological or relatively normal. One interesting possibility has to do with the instability in life circumstances that increasingly continues past adolescence into the twenties and even thirties, a phase some developmental psychologists have dubbed "emerging adulthood." The developmental psychologist Jeffrey Jensen Arnett, who pioneered the concept, has argued that significant substance use is normal at this developmental stage, as a means of seeking out new experiences before settling into adult life, but also as a way of dealing with the confusion inherent in settling on that stable adult identity.[11] If, as is often the case, meds complicate the process of figuring out who you are, then perhaps it's not surprising that young people on meds would be even more likely than their peers to seek either a kind of refuge or expanded self-awareness through substance use.

Yet I think it's fair to say that most of my medicated peers, even if they are peripherally aware that mixing substances is imprudent, don't see it as either a sign of dysfunction or a marker of being particularly unsure about their sense of self. As with rebellions against medication, drug or alcohol use in teenagers can be a way of resisting prescribed medications and the control they often represent—control that can feel oppressive and paternalistic to teens craving independence. As young people enter their late teens and twenties, combining nonprescribed substances with their medication becomes less about rebellion and more about proving that they can participate in the established social life of their peers, a social life that tends to involve a lot of drinking.

I've experienced this sentiment myself. When I was first prescribed Prozac at the end of high school and told not to drink because antidepressants could lower my tolerance and alcohol could interfere with the action of the meds, I dismissed the stricture as absurd—then paid for it with a case of near alcohol poisoning that I refused to connect to my medication. As I saw it, the point of taking Prozac in the first place was to allow me to function unencumbered by depression and anxiety, including in my social life. Shortly afterward, at a college whose unofficial motto was "Work hard, play hard," I considered my ability to party while taking antidepressants a sign of my competence. Even though I ended up a bit depressed, not to mention hungover, after a night out, I managed to earn top grades, participate enthusiastically in class discussions, throw myself into extracurriculars, offer support to friends, and have what I considered to be a full and satisfying college experience. When I briefly dated a boy who told me he couldn't drink heavily because alcohol interacted badly with his Zoloft, I considered him an unfortunate case, someone whose tenuous mental state and dependence on medication controlled his life in a way I refused to let it control mine.

A few people I interviewed, including Claire, tried to self-dose during college, avoiding meds on days they planned to drink heavily. (Claire, nervous about overburdening her body with too many pharmaceuticals, also tended to resist over-the-counter drugs like Tylenol.) But plenty of others exhibited a laissez-faire attitude toward substance use, ignoring the warning labels on their medication bottles. What medicine, after all, *doesn't* warn about combining it with alcohol? In some cases, familiarity with medication makes alcohol or illicit drugs seem less threatening. As one young woman with ADHD put it jokingly, "They tell me not to drive a car, operate machinery, drink alcohol, get pregnant, make conscious decisions. . . ." Her friend from high school, a young woman with a childhood history of intolerable side effects and ineffective meds, experienced black moods after drinking and smoking pot. She'd get down on herself, on life, sometimes on the efficacy of her antidepressant, which otherwise worked well for her. It took years before she could calmly remind herself that this grumpy, gloomy outlook wasn't cause for a crisis of confidence about her moods, her life, or her meds. Rather, it was the trade-off she had to make for partying—an emotional hangover.

Such partying habits don't sound excessive for someone in her late teens and early twenties, but having a history of stimulant use from childhood also raises another possibility that's perhaps more troubling than simply getting psychologically habituated to taking substances, whether prescribed or not. One of the longest-standing debates in child psychopharmacology concerns the impact of youth stimulant treatment on later substance abuse. Long-term studies published years ago found elevated rates of substance use in ADHD children as they grew up compared to kids who didn't have the disorder. But these studies often didn't take into account whether the children had been treated with stimulants. Doctors, parents, and researchers naturally began to wonder what role the drugs played—whether they reduced an already heightened tendency toward abusing substances, had no impact at all, or actually increased the risk by sensitizing reward pathways in the brain.

Animal studies show that rats exposed to a stimulant early in life become more sensitive to the rewards offered by other stimulants, such as cocaine, as they age. As more children began taking stimulants in the late 1980s and 1990s, the question loomed larger for parents, clinicians, and researchers, and scattered studies showed stimulant-treated kids were more prone to certain kinds of substance use later on, including cigarette smoking and cocaine use. In 2003, the eminent ADHD researcher Russell Barkley published the results of an influential, carefully designed thirteen-year study backing up the conclusions of eleven similar studies, which found "no compelling evidence that stimulant treatment of children with attention-deficit/hyperactivity disorder leads to an increased risk for substance experimentation, use, dependence, or abuse by adulthood."[12] Two studies from the National Institute on Drug

Abuse released in 2008 found stimulant-treated children weren't more likely to become drug addicts later in life.[13]

On an individual level, though, the pathways of causation can be maddeningly difficult to sort out because there are such high rates of comorbidity between psychiatric problems and substance-related problems. I interviewed a young man from northern California who was diagnosed with ADHD and medicated with stimulants at age five before cycling through several more diagnoses and classes of drugs and eventually being diagnosed with bipolar disorder. His parents monitored his medications carefully until he went away to college. Then, he decided to stop taking them because, he told me, "I wanted to trip harder on magic mushrooms." He discovered, to his disappointment, that clearing his system of psychiatric meds didn't, in fact, help him trip harder, so he began to drink more and more heavily, putting down a fifth of vodka a night with a couple of similarly inclined friends. He went back on medications a few months later, but continued to drink heavily and use cocaine. Did he abuse drugs and alcohol because stimulants sensitized the reward-seeking pathways in his brain? Perhaps his antipsychotics stopped working, leaving him vulnerable to mania, which is characterized by risky, pleasure-seeking behavior, including substance abuse. Or maybe after he quit his meds he began self-medicating to make up for their absence, and then continued to self-medicate when he got back on the drugs and they failed to get his moods in check. Did he have a comorbid substance use disorder, as do about half the people with bipolar disorder?[14] Or was he just having a particularly wild—and perhaps slightly belated—teenage rebellion? He couldn't begin to say.

Caleb, ages eighteen to twenty-two
TRI-CITIES, WASHINGTON / 2002–2006

During the most uncontrolled phases of his mania and mixed states, Caleb found his sense of reality shaken as though by an earthquake, his sense of himself and his emotions buried beyond his reach, as if by debris. Compared to the big, fundamental, philosophical questions about the nature of reality precipitated by his bipolar vacillations, heavy drinking was a more mundane but potentially important factor during both his decline and his recovery. In the months leading up to his near-suicide, he had been working long shifts on the catering staff of a local hotel, then embarking on crazy partying jaunts with his coworkers. Performing manual labor like that, moving tables and chairs for shifts that sometimes lasted fourteen hours at a stretch, he wanted something at the end of the day to ease the aches and pains, he told me. I can't help but think, though, that his need for release wasn't purely physical, that the quest for stimulation that so often characterizes mania played a role. He was the life of the party, and carried around a homemade beer funnel that could be employed for stunts as needed. His coworkers came from rough backgrounds—what Caleb described later as "the nooks and crannies of society"—and he found it refreshing that they didn't judge him at a time when he felt so alienated from much of his ordinary life. The "work hard, play hard" aspect of their lives appealed to him, too, especially in his manic phases. In the mixed states, or when he was simply too sore from hauling crates and furniture, alcohol, and sometimes some aspirin, took the edge off.

Heavy drinking and occasional pot smoking preceded his near-suicide attempt, and afterward his partying only intensified. At first, this was force of habit: he continued to work at the catering hall for a number of months, and, even after being fired, he still hung out with the friends he'd made there. But then he transferred to a four-year college upstate, where he continued to drink heavily, to do poorly in school, and to keep to himself, except when he went out dancing or was working as a nightclub bouncer. But within a few months, he began dating a young woman who drastically altered his outlook. Ever encouraging him, she made him believe, for the first time since his suicidal depression as a young teenager, that he could lead a stable and successful life. With this newfound peace of mind, small things started to satisfy him. He no longer had to go to extremes to feel something.

More candid than most of his peers, Caleb kept his psychiatrist apprised of his drinking. The psychiatrist didn't diagnose him with a substance use disorder, at least not that Caleb knew of, and I mention his partying not because it was so extreme, but rather because it is not atypical for his age group, and because it provides a useful example of the way substance use affects and complicates psychiatric diagnoses and treatment. Caleb and his psychiatrist might have interpreted his substance use in any number of ways. Was it a sign that he was incompletely recovered, and his medication ought to be adjusted further? A disorder in and of itself that required its own medication treatment? (Some psychotropic drugs, including Depakote, which he was prescribed as a mood stabilizer, are used to treat alcohol dependence.) An attempt to replicate the highs he had felt during the early parts of his manic phases? A reasonable and understandable attempt to connect with other people and his own emotions during a time when he was still feeling intensely alienated? A way to numb himself and to disguise the lingering numbness he felt after his breakdown? Or just an ordinary social activity for a twenty-something working a tiring, blue-collar job while also going to school, something that had nothing at all to do with his mood disorder or his treatment?

Caleb hadn't been prescribed medications carrying a high potential for abuse, such as stimulants for ADHD or antianxiety drugs. He didn't have to worry, then, about a potential consequence of being up front with his psychiatrist: the possibility that the doctor might decide to revoke an otherwise useful prescription because it might contribute to substance abuse. Teenagers and young adults have been under increasing scrutiny in recent years for abusing prescription drugs of various kinds, and, in particular, for abusing psychostimulants like Adderall, either to get high or party longer while drinking, or as study aids to increase concentration and alertness. (The subject has been discussed at length elsewhere, and I will deal with it here only briefly.) Government surveys show that young adults actually have higher reported rates of abusing psychotherapeutic drugs than teenagers do, with about 6 percent of young adults ages eighteen to twenty-five reporting doing so, versus 3 to 4 percent of adolescents.[15] Over the past fifteen years, the number of prescriptions for controlled substances written for young people has more than doubled, with stimulants being more commonly prescribed to teenagers and sedative/hypnotic drugs—sleeping meds and antianxiety meds—more commonly prescribed to young adults.

But none of these statistics tell us definitively whether young people are abusing their own prescriptions or whether they are giving or selling the meds to others.[16] The topic has been the subject of ample but inconclusive research, not to mention ongoing media coverage. It was even the subject of a 2007 film, *Charlie Bartlett*, about a teenager with ADHD who, courtesy of his prescription-happy psychiatrist, plays amateur psychopharmacologist to his high school. In my experience observing and interviewing, people tended to be more inclined to share or sell their stimulants or antianxiety drugs and, more rarely, sleeping meds, if the doctor prescribed far more than they needed or if they badly needed money. Usually, they didn't do so until after high school. Researchers who have studied college students' attitudes and habits regarding medication describe kids "prescribing" medications to their friends, often without bothering to figure out which drugs the friends might already be on.

Regardless of the particular numbers of young people abusing, trading, and selling meds, the subject has been in the public eye, and my peers and I are broadly aware of being scrutinized by doctors, family, and even friends in terms of our own use of prescription drugs. Some of us find the attention merely irritating, while others are acutely self-conscious of the way it exacerbates a sense of childishness and helplessness that comes with continuing psychiatric problems. Elizabeth, for example, was never vigilant about refilling prescriptions, in part because she feared doctors seeing her as dependent on a drug. With a family history of substance abuse and dependence, she had reason to worry. She tended to develop a rapid tolerance to Klonopin, her antianxiety drug, which rendered it less effective. Since much of her anxiety was tied up in her insomnia, she took Ambien for a time during her breakdown at college in California. She'd spend hours in a late-night haze before actually sleeping, dashing off incoherent and emotional e-mails to friends and boyfriends that often exacerbated the tension and melodrama that characterized many of her relationships and probably did little to calm her. Later, she concluded that Ambien was basically "drunk in a pill" and a poor choice for her, given her family history of alcoholism. Between her reluctance to ask for refills, her on-again, off-again attitude toward long-term antidepressant treatment, and the tendency for both Klonopin and Ambien to lose their effectiveness for her over time, Elizabeth's anxiety escalated so that, in the years after she flunked out of college, she often couldn't leave the house, make phone calls, or deal with other basic daily tasks. In not wanting to worry their psychiatrists about issues of addiction and dependence, people like Liz are then left to do the worrying on their own—yet more self-monitoring when, it seems, there is already so much to monitor.

Psychiatric disorders and their accompanying medication treatment are in one sense particularly impactful for young people because other health problems requiring ongoing medication are comparatively rare. The other maladies of youth are usually of short duration—broken bones, the flu, maybe mononucleosis. The chronic sports injuries I suffered in high school, and my childhood and teen experience with scoliosis, so visible and physically and psychologically restrictive, contrasted markedly with my medication treatment, which was invisible to my peers while feeling physically and psychologically liberating to me. There are, though, a handful of health complications that are likely to occur along with psychiatric disorders in young people—problems that intersect and interact with medication treatment and blur the boundary between the physical and the mental.

Migraines are worth singling out, because they occur about two to three times as often in people with mood and anxiety disorders as they do in the general population, and because their treatment often involves adding psychotropic drugs, or modifying existing drug regimens to accommodate other medications.[17] The headaches' peak onset is in the late teens and twenties, oftentimes, studies show, after psychiatric disorders have already manifested.[18] This means that young people may well be on medication before the headaches appear—and that when headaches do become problematic, treatment for them has to be worked into a drug regimen that already presents plenty of complications.

For frequent migraines, many of the preventive treatments of choice are psychotropic drugs, notably mood-stabilizing antiseizure meds and tricyclic antidepressants. In theory, treatment can kill two birds with one stone, but it can also interfere with one's existing psychotropic treatment. The triptan drugs prescribed to halt an acute headache in its tracks can interact dangerously with the SSRIs. Stimulants of various kinds are known to trigger headaches, and many doctors treating migraines advise not only against caffeine but also against ADHD medications.

Severe migraines may require someone already on medication to take yet another pill—often one that you've been previously unwilling to take. The sociologist David Karp says that people "carry around in their heads a kind of hierarchy of medications based on their relative acceptability."[19] The drugs used to treat more serious psychiatric disorders, such as schizophrenia and bipolar disorder, usually carry more of a stigma; they also tend to have more severe side effects. Beset by chronic migraines a decade after I had begun antidepressant treatment, I tried, in desperation, first one mood stabilizer and then another. Certainly, my situation was preferable to being diagnosed with epilepsy or bipolar disorder—two other conditions the mood stabilizers are used for—in which case I really would face the necessity of such drugs for life. But I resented the way that I'd now been forced to move into pharmaceutical territory I'd been lucky enough to avoid so far. The migraines also felt like a regression. Although I didn't feel the dizzy, nauseous, physical panic that had characterized my previous episodes of extended, intense anxiety, my neurologist suggested going back on Klonopin to control any latent stress and also avert the ever-present worry that a headache would worsen. My psychiatrist and therapist both agreed, though nobody seemed capable of explaining why my anxiety would now manifest as migraines, just as nobody had seemed capable of explaining why my teenage depression later manifested as anxiety. At twenty-eight, after more than a decade of treatment, I thought I knew myself well enough to recognize both anxiety and depression and know how my meds dealt with them. But now I felt outwitted.

Migraines are common before women have their periods, and severe PMS in general is also vastly more common among women with histories of anxiety and mood disorders. The reasons remain unclear. Researchers suspect that serotonin and other brain neurotransmitters interact with the changing levels of sex hormones. The result, though, is that even when a psychiatric disorder is under control, new mood symptoms often appear, or existing ones worsen with PMS. Whether to define severe PMS as its own psychiatric disorder—termed premenstrual dysphoric disorder, or PMDD, in an appendix of the *DSM-IV*—remains a matter of debate within the psychiatric profession and something of a trope among critics who argue that modern medicine, especially psychiatry, seeks to medicalize ordinary experience. Regardless of whether it should be considered its own disorder, though, the fact is that women with anxiety and mood disorders suffer from severe PMS at disproportionate rates.[20]

Regular PMS usually worsens with time, and several sources report the average age for the onset of PMDD as twenty-six. Here again is a condition that may well not appear until young women have already been taking psychotropic meds for years. After low-dose hormone birth control, SSRIs are considered first-line treatments; for women with mood and anxiety disorders, a higher dose may help with PMS. If that works, great. If not, the prognosis is complicated—notably for women with bipolar disorder, for whom antidepressants, even with the addition of a mood stabilizer, can trigger mania.

Many of the young women I interviewed said that they felt significantly worse around their periods but that they usually first attribute their symptoms to fights with friends, family, or significant others, troubles at school or work, juggling too many work or school projects, even a psychiatric relapse, before remembering that their periods are approaching. This is certainly common enough in women who don't take meds, but in those on long-term maintenance treatment this failure to see a connection between mood and biology is striking. If medications are effective, they work for the majority of the month to restore, or at least boost, the sense of competence and self-esteem that is so easily eroded by psychiatric problems. That a natural, biological event can temporarily—yet regularly—trump the effects of medication serves as a reminder of one's vulnerability.

Whereas low-dose hormone birth control pills and SSRIs are fairly well established treatments for severe premenstrual mood symptoms, the use of psychotropics during pregnancy and breast-feeding remains an area of intense research and few concrete answers. All psychotropic drugs cross the placenta and enter the blood circulating through the fetus; the extent to which they do so depends on the drug, the dosage, and the stage of pregnancy.[21] The FDA does not guarantee any psychotropics as safe during pregnancy. Rather, the agency rates them with a pregnancy warning system, as it does other classes of medication, according to their level of risk to the fetus. Most psychotropics are Class C, which indicates there is data from animal studies showing some level of increased risk to the fetus, or Class D, which indicates human data showing risk to the fetus.[22]

These choices and calculations of risk are not particular, of course, to the latest generation of women taking psychotropic medication. Since the new wave of psychopharmaceuticals began appearing in the late 1980s and prescriptions spiked, pregnant or would-be pregnant women have faced the prospect of balancing their own mental health and stability against the largely unknown risks to the fetus. The difference for me and my peers, compared to women facing this issue ten or twenty years ago, is that the magnitude and nature of the risks are somewhat better known, though far from conclusive, especially in regards to the long-term effects on children exposed to such drugs in the womb. More to the point, though, members of my generation of women were prescribed psychotropics at a younger age, when pregnancy wasn't even on their radar screens, or when they were primarily concerned only about *not* getting pregnant.

Upon becoming unintentionally pregnant a woman on medication can find herself in a situation even more fraught than that of the average young woman facing an unwanted pregnancy. In general, the fetus is most vulnerable during the first trimester because the most basic development of major systems occurs then—which means that women with unplanned pregnancies may have been taking psychotropic medications for many weeks before realizing they were pregnant. A young woman who had a diagnosis of bipolar disorder and had been taking a mood stabilizer described to me the process of learning she was pregnant and getting an abortion during college. She and her boyfriend agreed they simply weren't ready to raise a child—they had no money and they were in the middle of their educations. Knowing that the mood stabilizer she was taking had a high likelihood of causing birth defects or a miscar-

riage later on made the decision far easier: more objective, less emotional. She was only nineteen, and in her worldview and social circles,
an abortion was acceptable, even reasonable, under the circumstances.
Still, the experience made her think ahead to the children she knew she
wanted eventually. Her friends who weren't on heavy-duty medications
could comfort themselves with the assurances that someday, a decade or
so down the road, they could plan a pregnancy and do their utmost to
make it a healthy one, but she didn't see how that would be possible for
her, given doctors' prevailing wisdom for people with bipolar disorder:
don't go off your meds.

Indeed, pregnancy, as a period of shifting hormones, uncertainty,
and major life transition, is probably a particularly bad time to go courting relapse. One study showed that bipolar women were two and a half
times as likely to experience a relapse after going off their mood stabilizers during pregnancy as if they stayed on the drugs; another study of
women with histories of major depression found a similar likelihood
of relapse.[23] And these relapses can hurt not only the woman but the
child, should the mother incur dangerous risks while manic, or fail to
care for herself adequately while depressed. On the other hand, some
drugs, such as the atypical antipsychotics and lithium, carry physical
risks to the mother during pregnancy, such as high blood sugar, diabetes, and thyroid problems. Thinking ahead, this young woman who had
the abortion wasn't optimistic, though at nineteen she didn't see herself
starting a family for quite some time. In utero fetal risks created by the
atypical antipsychotics, the other major alternative to mood stabilizers, remain largely unknown.[24] Maybe they would be deemed safe by
the time this woman was ready to have children, or maybe not. For all
the advances in drugs to treat her condition, the desire to bear a child
someday left her feeling very much at a loss.

Claire, age thirty
KIRKLAND, WASHINGTON / 2010

In theory, women with psychiatric problems other than the disorders
involving mania and psychosis have a little more flexibility when it
comes to medications and pregnancy. Some of the most common drugs
used to treat depressive and anxiety disorders, the SSRIs and other anti-

depressants, have been shown to carry relatively little risk of serious birth defects (Paxil, which the FDA grades a Class D drug, seems to be an exception). But, as the psychiatry newsletter the *Carlat Psychiatry Report* put it in a 2010 review of the research, "whether they cause other problems such as preterm births or miscarriages is a matter of continuing debate."[25] The latest joint guidelines from the American Psychiatric Association and the American College of Obstetricians and Gynecologists recommended medication in a number of cases, including for women who, like Claire, have a history of severe, recurrent depression. The guidelines discourage use of Paxil but otherwise recommend a case-by-case approach to SSRI antidepressants, which can almost be more agonizing.[26]

Claire had begun treatment at eleven knowing, in theory, that she would likely need to take medications for the long haul; her parents presented her depression as treatable, but not curable—"a chemical imbalance" that needed ongoing calibration. Part of a large family, she wanted from childhood to have children of her own. Still, the possible risks of taking medications during pregnancy remained more or less the last thing on Claire's mind until her late twenties, when she married a video game developer she had met while teaching in the Bay Area. After they bought a house in the Seattle suburbs and began planning in earnest to have a child, the question of medication and pregnancy was hard to avoid. Her younger sister Bridget, also on psychotropic meds since middle school, had become a midwife who often counseled women about taking medication during pregnancy. Claire mined Bridget for information and combed popular websites and scientific articles for guidance. The evidence showed that various SSRIs had been associated with an increase in the risks of several serious but rare conditions— heart defects when taken early in pregnancy, a serious fetal lung condition when taken in the last half of pregnancy, skull malformations, a small intestine protruding from the belly button.[27] Claire knew that the risks of her baby developing any of these conditions remained very low, but the conditions sounded terrifying nonetheless.

She also knew if she stopped taking her meds, the odds of relapse were high. To cite just one example, a study of women with histories of depression and medication use estimated that those who discontinued medication were five times as likely to relapse as compared to women who maintained treatment. The study also found that having been on antidepressants for more than five years and having suffered four or more previous relapses increased the risk of relapse during pregnancy.[28] Both criteria applied to Claire, who had suffered two major relapses and numerous minor ones when on many occasions over the years her medications had ceased to work.

Bridget also warned about potential harm to the fetus should Claire relapse into depression or anxiety, a risk Claire's research confirmed. Indeed, anxious, depressed mothers are more prone to preterm birth and delivery complications. The negative effects of these mental disorders in pregnancy may delay infant development and persist well beyond infancy, resulting in lower academic achievement, greater emotional reactivity, and behavioral problems that may last through adolescence.[29]

Worried about relapse, Claire decided to take a middle route, by switching from Cymbalta, a newer drug with less information available about pregnancy outcomes, to Zoloft, for which there is more data showing that use during pregnancy carries minimal risks. The switch was hardly without sacrifice; Cymbalta, which she had been taking successfully for five years without its losing its efficacy the way her other meds had, had also been the one drug that hadn't left her exhausted during the daytime. Since the risks to the fetus are greatest during the first trimester, she switched medications before she and her husband began trying to have a child. She happened to make the switch when she was in the process of finishing up her job teaching middle school in the Bay Area prior to joining her husband in Seattle, where he had taken a new job.

When she had worked up to a therapeutic dose of Zoloft and found herself faring okay, she and her husband managed to conceive. However, she began spotting almost immediately and began to worry. She had a history of gynecological complications, including low levels of a hormone essential to maintain a pregnancy. At first she tried to minimize her fears, knowing how prone she was to anxiety. But as the bleeding grew worse, tests of her hormone levels revealed she was in danger of miscarrying. The doctors told her to go home and try to unwind, because stress could increase her likelihood of miscarriage. She'd taken

Klonopin in the past to control her anxiety, but the drug can cause severe birth defects, so she was left to her own devices. "Nothing like knowing your unborn child's life is on the line to help a girl decompress," she noted, with her characteristic sarcasm, on the blog she had started for pregnant women with depression. When her hormone levels continued to drop, the miscarriage was assured. She continued to bleed for a month and slept on towels, so as not to ruin the couple's brand-new sheets. She also fell into a deep depression, which she interpreted thus: "It wasn't the broken-hearted, 'I am an empty shell without my beloved child' unhappiness that I had seen on movies. I was only pregnant a few weeks. No, this was the despondent, lonely, disassociated, broken-hormone stuff that comes with clinical depression. It sucked." When she wasn't working at a local tutoring center, she stayed home and sobbed, in the helpless way of very bad PMS. Logically, she knew that she could just as soon get pregnant again or, that failing, she and her husband could adopt. She didn't ponder the loss of life, or the possibility of being unable to pass on her genes to her child. It reminded her of the times in high school when her medication had stopped working, and she had been too depressed to take a shower.

Upon moving to Seattle, Claire had chosen a psychiatrist who specialized in medications during pregnancy, and she now recommended that Claire switch back to Cymbalta at least until she stabilized. After the worst of the cramping and bleeding stopped, her mood improved—a combination, Claire thought, of the switch in medication and her hormones returning to normal. Reminded of the awfulness of a truly deep depression, Claire gave thanks that medication had pulled her out and decided to remain on it at least until she got pregnant again. As Claire told me, half joking, a few months later, despite her husband's superhuman patience, if she stayed a volatile, weepy, cranky mess the prospect of even getting to the point of potential conception was highly unlikely.

She conceived a second time a couple of months later. Still, she worried about maintaining the pregnancy and remained conflicted about her meds, as antidepressants can increase the risk of miscarrying. Her doctors' uncertainty and lack of ready answers—about miscarrying, about her mental health—wore on her increasingly. She thought back to her childhood pediatrician who first diagnosed her depression and prescribed medication. He seemed "so composed, collected, and spoke with such certainty that I suspect he got all his information directly from God." She and her husband had discussed the possibility of her going off medications for the duration of the pregnancy, quitting her tutoring job, and just staying home, waiting out the pregnancy. But that seemed certain to stimulate a relapse—being home alone, isolated, with nothing to do with herself.

In the end, her psychiatrist put an end to her indecision by recommending she at least try going off her Cymbalta for the remainder of her first trimester, when the risk of miscarriage is highest. Claire decided to give it a shot and began tapering down her dose to half. But as she began spotting again, and worrying about the results from her latest hormone tests to see if she would be able to maintain the pregnancy, her anxiety spiked. In the past Claire's depression had often culminated in fits, but this one was a standout, complete with screaming, wailing, hyperventilating, dripping snot all over, dry heaving. Unlike when she received the news of her first miscarriage and fell into a month-long depression she dismissed as purely hormonal, she interpreted this meltdown as a clear reaction to the stress and uncertainty of her situation. As she put it, "There is nothing like being unsure whether or not your child is actually dying inside you: the massive disappointment, the feelings of inadequacy, and helplessness; it's unreal." Angry at herself for not being able to keep it together, she decided to return to the full dose of her meds. Considering her track record, the stress didn't seem worth the small risks to the baby, or the increased risk of postpartum depression after she delivered. She decided to wait and see.

CHAPTER 9

Reassessments

*When I say that I will be on medication indefinitely, people who have dealt
calmly and sympathetically with the news of suicide attempts,
catatonia, missed years of work, significant loss of body weight,
and so on stare at me with alarm.*

—ANDREW SOLOMON, *The Noonday Demon*

Andrew Solomon's sweeping and acclaimed "atlas of depression" was
published more than a decade ago, and in a short section of a very long
book he recounts that since he is writing a book on depression, people
often ask him to describe his own experience. He usually concludes by
saying that he is on psychotropic drugs, which invites well-meaning
but ultimately patronizing lectures about the risks of taking long-term
medications. I find his description of people's reactions striking because
when I talk about my book and mention I have taken medication since
adolescence, most people don't question my experience of medication
but instead want to know what conclusions I come to in the book. Are
kids, in fact, overmedicated? Is growing up on meds good or bad for
people? Are there long-term physical or psychological side effects?

I suspect their reaction results from the generalizing and polemi-
cal ways in which we, as a society, tend to discuss psychiatric medication, especially for children and teenagers. Everyone, it seems, already
has an opinion—and they want to know how my opinion compares to

theirs. I try to summarize what I've learned in the process of writing this book—that it's not so simple as meds being good or bad for young people in general; that the long-term side effects remain largely unknown but that large longitudinal studies are under way; and, most of all, that the psychological impact of the experience varies vastly from person to person, depending on his or her upbringing, personality, present circumstances, and inherited predisposition to illness. Certainly, for people of any age, the combination of having diagnosed psychiatric problems and an ongoing medication regimen that alters their moods, behavior, and thought processes poses a potentially serious challenge to their sense of self, a phenomenon that psychiatrist Peter Kramer explored nearly twenty years ago in *Listening to Prozac*, and that numerous bioethicists and other scholars have examined since. When these phenomena converge with all the rapid changes inherent in growing up, the process of understanding one's disorder, one's medication, and oneself—both separately and also in concert—becomes far more difficult.

Clearly, the question of young people and medication is a pressing issue, and people want and need guidance. Each of my subjects has struggled, and continues to struggle, with his or her own demons. Since medical science still does not entirely understand how psychotropic medications work to relieve symptoms, the process of prescribing and using them is less like a mathematical equation than a process of trial and error. What works, or seems to work, for any particular patient in a given set of circumstances may not work for the same patient or another patient facing a different set of challenges. Ongoing longitudinal studies may clarify some of the larger unresolved medical questions over the next decade or two, but researchers are unlikely to be able to provide a definitive treatment protocol that will work for every patient at every stage in life. Personalized treatments using biomarkers are still far from being available for clinical practice.

Interviewing my peers has convinced me that even young people with long histories of medication use haven't fully processed their experiences. The subjects featured or quoted in this book agreed to talk to me because they found something compelling in my premise that medication has shaped who they are, who they seem to be, or who they declare themselves to be. Although the five young people whose stories I have told in depth were often stymied by my questions, they gamely tried to give me the answers that seemed right for them at that moment, and they continued to refine, elaborate, and revise their answers over the two to three years that I interviewed them. Of course, it's impossible to do justice to the full texture of their current situations or to their individual assessments of what medication has meant for them over the course of their lifetimes. But it is nevertheless worth a look at where they are now, how they judge their journeys thus far, and how they imagine their futures vis-à-vis medication.

Claire, age thirty-one
KIRKLAND, WASHINGTON / 2011

At nearly eight months pregnant, Claire had remained on her full, pre-pregnancy dose of Cymbalta after she experienced a depressive meltdown while trying to taper off in her first trimester. During that meltdown, she had felt "possessed" and, looking back on it, horrified, as she always was when she considered her breakdowns in hindsight. Despite continuing medication, toward the end of her pregnancy she could feel her depression returning, though she sounded cheery as ever when I spoke with her. Her posts on Facebook—about the baby's sonogram, the fleece booties she knitted and the quilt she made, the nursery furnishings her mother and mother-in-law sent—seemed as full of excitement and anticipation as those of any expectant mother. Her psychiatrist had mentioned that her dose might not be as effective now that her blood volume had increased so much, but she also attributed her creeping unhappiness to isolation, as the tutoring center where she worked had been reducing her hours in anticipation of her departure when the baby was born. Her younger sister, who had also been taking psychotropic meds since early adolescence, was suffering a protracted relapse, and that wore on Claire, too, though everyone told her not to worry since stress was bad for the baby.

Until her eighth month, she had been planning to remain on Cymbalta throughout her pregnancy and afterward, but her research showed that babies born to mothers who had taken the drug in late pregnancy often suffered withdrawal symptoms at birth, and that the drug is particularly likely to be transmitted through breast milk. As a result, she was considering going off drugs altogether, then possibly switching back to Zoloft for breast-feeding. She didn't frame it as such, but to me going off Cymbalta sounded like a major sacrifice: on medication almost continuously for two decades, she doesn't recognize herself when they stop working, or when she misses doses for too long. "The person who I am when I'm off my medication, that's not me—that's someone else," she had told me. She was speaking to me and her husband, who began antidepressant treatment in his twenties and considers it a choice to enhance his well-being, not a necessity. He thinks he is more himself without the drugs, but that they make him a better person. Claire's choice is starker. "If I want to remain who I am," she said, "then I need to take my medication."

Having suffered a deep depression following her miscarriage, which she attributed to massive hormonal shifts, she was, despite considering stopping meds for the final weeks of her pregnancy, deeply worried about postpartum depression. Isolation, she suspected, and the lack of sleep having a new baby entails, would likely only worsen her moods. "I've wanted a baby since I was like nine," she told me, "and what I'm terrified of is that I will have one and I will be miserable. But," she added, "my mom assures me that I'm so sensitive to all those hormones—like all those love hormones that will be raging around—that I'll be all right."

Still, aware of the ample body of research showing poorer emotional outcomes for infants of depressed mothers, she wanted to do everything she could to avoid depression. Having learned from experience to put the necessary supports in place to guard against relapse before it arrived, she joined a support group for women at risk of postpartum depression. For the first time in a decade, she has entered therapy, despite continuing doubts about how effective it would be for her, wry, straightforward, and literal-minded as she is. She let the therapist, a former midwife, know when it got to be "too much therapy," like the time the woman asked, "What kind of messages are you getting right now from your baby?" "I dunno," Claire deadpanned. "The conversation has been kind of one-sided."

With twenty years of antidepressants under her belt, she has retained the same core attitudes about treatment: a conviction about the need for long-term maintenance medication for her depression and anxiety, tempered with frustration with certain side effects and the drugs' inability to treat some symptoms. She wishes she'd learned more techniques to both recognize and cope with her anxiety when she was younger; the emphasis was on her depression diagnosis and on meds, though she notes that at the time she was lucky to have gotten a diagnosis at all. When she was a kid she thought less about how her depression and her treatment affected others; her parents "kind of made their living with that stuff," and her siblings were hardly her top concern. Now that she's older and preparing to give birth, she thinks about how her condition affects her husband, her child, and her other relationships. "It makes it kind of a bigger deal because it is not just about me anymore," she says. "Now it is more of a responsibility thing. I can't be lazy and shrug it off if I skip my meds one day, or my meds aren't *quite* right, or have a weird sleepy side [e]ffect. I have to be really good about keeping all of this under control because it affects those I love, who are ultimately more important to me than I am to myself."

She often thought about the prospect of her daughter developing a mental illness, given that it was prevalent on both sides of her family, and that her husband had experienced depression requiring medication in his twenties. As she pondered the possibility, she was grateful she'd had the chance to analyze her own experience so carefully from childhood on. With everything she has experienced and seen in her own family, she's confident she knows what to look for and when to intervene—with meds if necessary.

Paul, age twenty-three
FORT LAUDERDALE, FLORIDA / 2011

Paul, now twenty-three, is enrolled in college in Fort Lauderdale, and works several jobs. He has not taken psychotropic medications in years—since he quit secretly at age sixteen. Shortly before he turned eighteen, he "came out" with his desire to be off the meds for good, and after consulting Paul's foster-care caseworker about how he had been faring without his meds, Paul's psychiatrist did not represcribe. Paul's own view of his treatment seems inextricably bound up with his feelings of neglect both before and after he entered the foster-care system, as well as the way in which he was left completely on his own at age eighteen. (He graduated high school while living in a homeless shelter, where he spent six months before an evangelical Christian church admitted him to a home for foster children aging out of the system.) On a church-led service trip to the Bahamas, Paul toured an orphanage where the children, dressed in rags and without toys, struck him as immeasurably happier than he himself had felt or his foster-care peers in Fort Lauderdale had seemed. As far as he could tell, none of the Bahamian orphans were taking psychiatric drugs (though he didn't specifically inquire). Increasingly, his own experience with medication seemed an inappropriate patch for behavior problems that stemmed from a fundamental, but not psychiatric, problem: his intense desire for a caring, loving, stable home and family. Several years later, he worked at one of the group homes where he had lived as a young teen, and decided that many of the kids were disturbed enough to need medication. But he maintains that in his case, the meds were wrongly prescribed. "The point is, medication never did anything for me," he said. "Never did I feel like a loose cannon." He thinks the Florida foster-care system in general has medicated far too many children. Though he always insisted to me that he was in control of his behavior, caseworkers and psychologists whom I spoke with insisted that he was a charismatic but uncontrollable little boy who posed a real threat to himself and others. He seemed to suffer not only from a grave lack of love and stability, but from an inability to verbalize his feelings. Since then, he has given up his tough-guy posturing and become far more comfortable and adept at discussing what's inside.

His faith in God, which intensified after he aged out of the system, and his church, a mega-congregation of twenty thousand close to his home in Fort Lauderdale that is part of a network of more than a thousand affiliated churches worldwide, seem to have helped him by providing the comfort, love, and support he lacked as a child and teenager. His experience being medicated against his will has also determined his current emphasis on the importance of what the Bible calls loving-kindness. "It did shape my view of the world—how the world values things that don't belong," he told me. People don't value something that doesn't belong to them or isn't their responsibility. So you see the world isn't as compassionate as it should be." It's clear he is struggling to heal wounds from both before and after he entered the foster-care system, in part by devoting much of his time and attention to organizations involving foster children. He serves as a residential advisor in a house for foster children aging out of the system and has worked for years at an emergency shelter not unlike the one where he stayed upon being taken from his parents. He is engaged to a young woman who had a child as an unwed teen mother, and can't wait to form a family with her and her two-year-old daughter. He has found mentors and forged important contacts with adults who help him in myriad ways. Meanwhile, he is working as a busboy in the restaurant of a Miami hotel and doesn't expect to finish school until 2013. In his current zest for life and flurry of commitments, it is hard to tell how much he is just trying to make up for what he missed and how much he is still struggling.

Alex, age twenty-three
BROOKLYN, NEW YORK / 2011

Alex, who is enrolled in a medieval history master's program and has self-published four works of Catholic philosophy, remains on medication, which he credits with helping him stabilize his depression and anxiety, but not with doing away with his obsession with his former classmate. He has endured a long and fraught recovery after quitting his medication in frustration and sinking into a rapid and deep depression in early 2010. But his drug regimen of the last eighteen months has stabilized his moods and helped him "be the person I'm supposed to be." The meds have not entirely transformed him into that person; rather, he thinks, they have primed him for more productive self-examination and self-understanding.

From the time he began taking medication at age ten, Alex has combined drug treatment with therapy. At present, he places considerable emphasis on his decision to abandon the counselor who wanted him to pursue a relationship with another man. Whereas his previous therapists practiced cognitive-behavioral therapy in the hope of controlling his inclination toward anxiety, depression, and obsession, his current psychiatrist has focused on the role Alex's upbringing—specifically his absent father and deeply strained relationships with his mother's two other serious lovers—has played in his behavior, thoughts, and emotions.

Six months after resuming the meds, Alex had a therapeutic revelation: when people were mean to him, it was as much about their own problems as about him. As he put it, "I realized that people were not deliberately trying to hurt me. It's just that they do not have it in them to be any better than they are, and would still be bad even if I was not around." While this improved his self-esteem, it also caused him to adopt an even more stridently misanthropic pose. Then, nine months after the breakthrough, he decided to become a more devout Catholic and noticed feeling less misanthropic, less tempted to overeat, and less attracted to other men. Crucially, he came to a new understanding of his obsession with his former classmate; he says his mother "cracked the case." What he'd thought was a sexual and romantic attraction was merely an emotional identification with a boy who, Alex recently confirmed, has family problems of his own. Alex now thinks that the rejection was devastating mostly because it symbolized all the rejections by the other men in his life—his absent, and then deceased, father, and his mother's two boyfriends, the second of whom became his stepfather. Yet, having come to this conclusion, he continued to think about the boy, though not so relentlessly. At the time of this writing, he was trying to relax and waiting to see where the thoughts might lead him.

Alex never committed to medication unequivocally, but since his breakdown after high school, he has rejected his stepfather's view that medication, especially for psychiatric problems, represents weakness. He bases that primarily on his own experience, but he notes that his stepfather's attitude may have ultimately been his undoing: having continued to shun his epilepsy medications, he died of a seizure-induced heart attack in 2008.

Except for the two weeks in late 2009 when he quit in frustration over the medications' lack of effects, Alex has pragmatically accepted his need to take the drugs, which have, for the most part, gotten him through the worst times. Nonetheless, he retains a nugget of the ambition common to so many people who take psychiatric drugs, whatever their age: to be free of medication eventually. He can't articulate why; he doesn't even notice any side effects. Nonetheless, his newfound self-acceptance and self-understanding, combined with the recent improvement in his mood and the diminishing of his obsessional thoughts, have given him hope that he can begin tapering off the meds, carefully, sometime in the next year or so.

Caleb, age twenty-seven
AUSTIN, TEXAS / 2011

Caleb has remained on mood-stabilizing and antidepressant medication continuously since his bipolar diagnosis at age nineteen. After three years in community college and three more at a state school a couple hours from his hometown, he graduated college with a major in technical communications. Since then, he has lived in Austin, Texas, where he splits his time between freelance gigs in the technology and creative fields. Setting his own schedule suits him. His medications disrupt his sleep schedule; he also chafes at the strictures of a nine-to-five job. That the medications not only kept him alive but also allowed him to graduate college and function independently in the world is, he says, a miracle. As he puts it, "I have not been able to hold a steady job for any corporate people, that's a little beyond my reach. But I might be able to live in the world. That's kind of what I'm trying to do now." His parents pay for his health-care costs out of pocket—buying individual insurance is too costly—but now that he has stabilized on meds, he sees his psychiatrist only every nine months for refills and buys generic drugs in bulk from Walmart.

Caleb has the ability to accommodate what seem like contradictory perspectives. I can't help but think it may be part of having come back to midpoint after the highs of mania and the lows of depression. He is at once strikingly generous to and sharply critical of the mental health profession, thanking his therapists and psychiatrists for "doing the best with the information they had" but also delivering a withering critique of the methods used to diagnose people and determine treatment. The son of a scientist, he is angrily dissatisfied with the state of the science of drug development. He advocates the radical-sounding solution that patients experiment with new treatments on themselves. As he puts it, "If something doesn't exist with computers, you build it. It gets built overnight." Yet, unlike so many others, he doesn't blame pharmaceutical companies: naturally, they are going to go where the profits are, which consists of tweaking competitors' drugs and marketing their existing portfolio for new uses. Caleb sees himself in a category apart from a general group of people who take medication for less severe mood problems, and yet he hesitates to "diagnose" individuals based on his own observations, as I and others are so prone to do. "I've been to places where I guess people would think was very scary, so to me maybe things are more extreme. I've been on medicine for so long, I don't know what normal is anymore."

Elizabeth, age thirty
WASHINGTON, DC, SUBURBS / 2011

For much of the past two years, psychiatric medications have, curiously, been somewhat on the back burner for Elizabeth—and not because she has figured out her drug regimen, or her attitudes toward medication treatment in general. Rather, she was diagnosed with an autoimmune thyroid disorder and an associated tumor. The former is notorious for mimicking the symptoms of mania, anxiety, and depression. Her focus shifted from trying to find the perfect cocktail of psychiatric meds to finding the right cocktail of thyroid medication and arranging to have the tumor removed. That has proved enormously difficult. Already devastated by her mother's sudden death in 2007, the latest diagnoses, though they seemed to explain some of her wildest moods, have also thrown her into an even greater tailspin. She has not returned to school or been able to work. Her father, from whom she is estranged, pays for her health insurance premiums and copayments, and she pays for other expenses with her inheritance from her mother.

As Liz often points out, her experience demonstrates the way in which the brain-body dichotomy so many people subscribe to can be misleading and damaging. Although her ADHD and anxiety showed up in elementary school, and depression in middle school, likely long before her thyroid condition developed, she has never been so disturbed or disturbing as when her thyroid is in overdrive. Apart from contributing to her ongoing academic turmoil, the hyperthyroid episodes have caused her sister to stop speaking to her and have ruined two serious romantic relationships in two years. Recently, when the thyroid medications were not working properly, she began cutting herself again and, for the first time ever, having suicidal thoughts. "It seems like once you are being treated for something psychological, medical doctors stop looking for medical explanations for symptoms and start writing you off as someone who just needs to see a psychiatrist instead," she says. "I think for most of my life we've been using medication to treat a lot of symptoms that were almost certainly caused by my thyroid disorder." By temporarily and partially treating the symptoms, the psychotropic drugs, she thinks, delayed getting to the root cause of many of her problems.

A psychology major in college and avid reader of anything on the subject, Liz has become a largely self-taught expert on mental illness. Her openness about her own medication use has over the years resulted in many friends and acquaintances opening up about their experiences. Once ready to chew out anyone who disparaged her for taking medication, she has herself grown increasingly wary of psychotropics, though she calls them "a useful tool." In 2009, a friend who was depressed, but not deeply, committed suicide after being badly sick with the flu and vomiting up his Zoloft for days. Zoloft has a short half-life, and Liz has experienced withdrawal from the drug several times. She thinks being rapidly deprived of Zoloft probably contributed to his suicide. She wonders, too, if when she cut herself in high school after going off Prozac, it was not a relapse, but withdrawal.

Her doctor assures her that when her thyroid is removed and her hormone treatment worked out, her mood problems could resolve, but she suspects she'll probably continue to need psychotropic meds indefinitely. Yet, between side effects and safety concerns, she says, "I'm probably never going to find the magical 'right' balance of medications that I can stay on long term and do well on."

Although I am not a mental health professional or an expert in child development, my work on this book has revealed certain circumstances that are likely to make the experience of taking medication during one's formative years easier to navigate.

Kids fare better when they understand the need for medications, either because they themselves perceive something wrong with their moods or behavior, or because parents and doctors do a good job of explaining why the meds are necessary and what the child can reasonably expect. They also do better when adults take seriously children's concerns and opinions about medication, not just at the outset but throughout treatment, and when children understand that psychiatric meds aren't akin to a course of antibiotics but require extended use. Kids do better when they trust their prescribing doctor and when the doctor makes clear why it's important to take the meds as prescribed and not to stop them abruptly or secretly. They do better when parents gradually give them more responsibility for their own treatment as they move through adolescence, rather than leaving them entirely to their own devices, as Elizabeth's parents did, or controlling treatment completely until some arbitrary point and then checking out altogether, as the foster-care system effectively did for Paul.

The data also show that for most conditions, kids do better, as do adults, with combined medication and therapy, although a dwindling number of psychiatrists provide both, and most insurance companies severely limit their coverage of therapy. Even when kids are fortunate enough to receive both forms of treatment, they typically don't have an opportunity to discuss how they actually feel about their medications. Despite all the factions and splits among mental health professionals, I think it's fair to say that most of them subscribe to some variation of the so-called biopsychosocial model, which recognizes the complicated and largely unknown interplay of genetic, environmental, social, and psychological factors in the development and course of psychiatric disorders. But clinicians are still far less attuned to what a few psychiatrists have wisely called "the psychology of psychopharmacology," the ways in which the experience of taking medications influences kids. In practice, usually, the drugs are the realm of the prescribing doctor while everything else is relegated to the therapist, or a psychiatrist conducts traditional therapy sessions and hurriedly inquires about meds at the end of the appointment. Yet, studies show that a strong therapeutic relationship is important not only to adherence but to the efficacy of the pill itself.[1] I'm not suggesting that doctors or therapists should plumb for meaning or symbolism in medication where there is none. But even if kids don't conceive of the medication shaping their overall outlook in life, doctors and therapists should help their patients understand that medication is not, in most cases, a quick fix.

The vast majority of parents only want what's best for their sons and daughters, but they need to talk to their kids—and observe them carefully—because they can't presume to know every contour of their children's emotional landscapes, either before medication or afterward. Research demonstrates that parents very often underestimate or fail to notice at all when children are suffering from internalizing disorders such as depression and anxiety. Externalizing, or behavioral, disorders, moreover, can obscure the feelings and motivations beneath. Children and teens, meanwhile, can be enormously secretive; they also often assume their parents see and know far more than they do. Meeting with Caleb and his parents, for example, I was struck by how much his parents' perceptions differed from his: where they had seen an unhappy young teen, Caleb had seen no point in living, and later, where he had experienced the mile-a-minute pace of mania, they had seen nothing awry. Even Claire's parents, as her mother made a point of emphasizing to me, largely missed the signs of depression—not just in Claire but in two siblings diagnosed afterward, despite her father's personal history and professional experience with mental illness. And many young people treated for ADHD, including Elizabeth, described their intense wish that they could control their tempers and focus their attention, even as their parents took their outbursts and lack of focus as rebelliousness, or as lack of commitment or ambition.

These communication gaps may well continue, or even widen, once kids get medication. Parents may conclude that by getting their children on medication and seeing a doctor, they have dealt with the problem, as Liz eventually concluded her parents had done. Medication, even when it works to reduce symptoms, creates its own questions and problems, which themselves evolve as kids mature and their circumstances and outlooks change.

Inviting kids' opinions about their medication treatment and giving them more say in their care as they mature is important not only because it makes it less likely that children will rebel against the meds, and, in turn, resent their parents and doctors; it is also important because it helps prepare them to make wise decisions about their treatment as they transition to adulthood. When patients have continuing psychiatric problems, ongoing drug treatment may be warranted—or it may not be. But young people with a history of medication should at least be aware of how their experiences have shaped their attitudes toward meds so that they can make those decisions for the right reasons, not to settle a score or to compensate for a bad experience.

Liz's case, which includes difficult-to-treat physical health problems and little social or family support, is especially complicated. She often seemed to me in a perpetual maelstrom of problems that made it difficult to prioritize and make even the smallest steps toward stabilizing. That was also true of some other people I interviewed with severe and intractable mental illnesses that did not respond to medication. But even medicated young people with more easily treated conditions face many logistical treatment hurdles as they transition to adulthood. Results from a large federal survey of mental health service use found, for example, that young people aged eighteen and nineteen use services at about half the rate of teens aged sixteen and seventeen and that rates remained low through age twenty-five. After age eighteen significantly fewer youths had services covered by private insurance and many more paid out of pocket or relied on charity care.[2] Young adults are less likely to have health insurance than other age groups. Recent data shows that the percentage of uninsured among young adults aged nineteen to thirty-four is nearly double the national average and nearly three times that of children, who are more likely to be covered either by their parents' health plans or by public insurance. The majority of these uninsured young adults work full-time, but are far more likely than older workers to be in jobs without employer-sponsored coverage.[3] Clearly, this is a larger structural problem. The health-care reform bill of 2010 sought to remedy the lack of coverage by requiring employers to provide coverage for employees' dependent children through age twenty-six, rather than cutting them off at age eighteen or nineteen, as many states had previously allowed. Starting in 2014, most everyone will be required to buy insurance or pay a penalty, although as of this writing there were numerous pending court challenges.

Part of the motivation behind the bill lay in the benefits of insuring as many people as possible; by requiring everyone to carry insurance, it will also ensure that the "young and healthy" pay premiums that subsidize the care of the older and sicker. The fact remains, however, that most young adults can, depending on their tolerance for risk, get away without insurance altogether or with the cheapest, most basic coverage; some have argued that paying the fine would be cheaper than complying with the mandate. My medicated peers and I can't afford to cut these corners, though. We need plans with good prescription drug coverage and good mental health benefits. Finding those plans at an affordable price is difficult, especially in an adverse job market. Those with more serious conditions who lack coverage must pay very high out-of-pocket costs for doctor's visits and prescriptions. Some simply stop taking their meds, thereby courting relapse and maybe hospitalization, the most expensive and drastic option of all.

Those with less disabling symptoms still may be psychologically reliant on knowing they can continue to take their medications, or at least resume taking them should they begin to function poorly again. Their need for particular insurance benefits can limit their job choices, which can have serious implications for their career options for years to come. Many have no choice but to take jobs that require them to pay high, ongoing out-of-pocket medical costs. People I interviewed described paying as much as $1,200 a month for medications and doctor's copayments. One young woman I interviewed, who had been diagnosed with bipolar disorder by several doctors, described applying for a managerial position at the cell phone customer service call center where she worked, not because she wanted to be a manager—she liked working directly with customers—but because she needed the mental health benefits. At the time, her outlays on her mental health were $500 a month. Even after taking the managerial position, she continued to worry that a relapse would get her fired and she would lose her medical benefits.

Some parents who can afford it are willing to help pay insurance premiums or copays, but this places a huge burden on them, inspires guilt or feelings of inadequacy in kids, and creates tensions between both parties. Another young woman I interviewed, who had been diagnosed with bipolar disorder and Asperger's syndrome, had been on a raft of medications since adolescence. She had fifteen psychiatrists in eleven years, mostly because of insurance issues. When I first spoke to her, she had recently filed for federal disability status because her father, who had been paying for her insurance premiums, had fallen badly ill, stopped working, and gone on disability himself. Liz's father pays for health insurance, but he won't pay out of pocket for out-of-network therapy. She has been able to work just six months in the past decade. Caleb's parents pay his health-care costs, but they worry about how long they will have to do so.

Beyond the cost and logistical hurdles involved in securing adequate insurance coverage and treatment, young adults face problems with continuity of care. The medical profession tends to bifurcate into pediatricians and psychiatrists who treat children and adolescents, and general practitioners and psychiatrists who treat adults. Child and adolescent psychiatrists are also certified to treat adults, but unless a clinician has formed a particular bond with a patient, treatment usually ends around the time kids reach eighteen, or move away from home. I interviewed one person who had lived in the same town and continued to see the same doctor for her whole life, but the days when people remain in the same town with the same family doctor are mostly gone. Young adults are a particularly mobile group, bouncing from city to city, state to state, job to job, school to job and back to school; young adults with psychiatric problems tend to be even more unsettled than their peers.

Even if they manage to maintain insurance coverage throughout, they often see multiple prescribing doctors, often for only brief periods of time. My own life has been relatively stable, but due to the usual moving around, I have had somewhere between seven and nine doctors prescribing my meds in ten years. Oftentimes they prescribed a nine-month supply, and I took large stashes with me when I did internships or study abroad programs, or moved someplace new and took my time finding a new psychiatrist. Many of the people I interviewed said they had no idea how many doctors they've seen.

Yet it's the rare person who bothers to have his records transferred to each and every new physician, and also the rare person who keeps his own records of medications and dosages—though that would certainly be a good idea (I am a careful record keeper in general, yet I remember being stunned when, a few years back, a psychiatrist suggested I do so for my medications). The vast majority of people I interviewed said they couldn't recall the specific details of their medication histories, itself "a very disempowering feeling," one young woman said. Since, for the reasons explained in my introduction, my subject base is likely skewed toward those with more serious or intractable conditions, they have probably cycled through more drugs than the average medicated young person. But even those with fairly limited psychiatric histories often can't recall dosages, or how long they were on a given drug, or even what side effects prompted them to switch one drug for another. Serious episodes of mental illness, furthermore, wreak havoc on one's memory while they last; people remember some details with acute vividness and others not at all. To compound the problem, some drugs, like the short-acting antianxiety agents in the benzodiazepine class of drugs, interfere with the formation of new memories.[4] The younger people were when they began treatment, the hazier all this gets. Some parents keep good rec-ords themselves. Most think that's the doctor's job.

Doctors consider medical histories important in making prescribing decisions; that's why they have you fill out detailed forms at your first visit and why psychiatrists usually spend a lengthy initial session doing an "intake" exam to go over the patient's history. Ideally, they should know which drugs, and at which dosages and in which combinations with other drugs, have or have not worked in the past, and have or have not caused particular side effects. And, if they are to be at all useful in providing a sounding board for a patient's concerns about medications—something I believe is very important, given how uncommonly the topic is discussed even with close friends—they ought to know at least the basic outlines of one's medical history. The bottom line: parents should keep detailed records of their child's prescriptions, dosages, and side effects until a child is ready to do it for herself.

Along with these pressing logistical hurdles, young adults face philosophical challenges as they take control over their own treatment. Among the most vexing decisions, I think, is how much to disclose about one's current medication use and past history. Typically, the decision is not very much, even in a culture where medications are much discussed in the abstract. Young adults just starting out in their careers are understandably wary about revealing their psychiatric history to employers and face a quandary regarding medications: they are afraid their reliance on psychotropic drugs could adversely affect their chances of getting a job or being promoted to a position of greater responsibility, but they are also aware that disclosing their decision to stop taking medication may raise doubts about their competence and judgment.

    For a generation immersed in the language and psychology of the psychopharmaceutical revolution and accustomed to disclosing the most personal information on public or semi-public media platforms, members of my cohort are surprisingly close-mouthed about our psychiatric medications, except in the "safe" settings of support groups, pseudonymous online forums, or with friends who share similar problems. The stigma of ongoing psychiatric difficulties, as opposed to transient, passing concerns, remains potent. It's one thing to disclose, conspiratorially and in the proper company, that you currently have a prescription for Adderall or Xanax to get you through a stressful period, or to say in passing, "Oh, yeah, I tried Zoloft for a while in high school, but I didn't like how it made me feel," or, "I took Ritalin for ADHD when I was a kid, but I grew out of it." But to confess to being someone who has, as Lauren Slater put it in *Prozac Diary*, "with great consideration, tied the slow satin knot" of commitment to long-term treatment is to put oneself in a very different category.[5] In my experience, people don't usually respond with the preachy tone Andrew Solomon describes encountering when he confesses to indefinite treatment. But they do tend to make judgments nonetheless—they may concede, for example, that while bipolar disorder and schizophrenia require lifelong treatment and are severely impairing, most anything else is conquerable by other means, and that medication is an easy way out.

There can be more tangible and serious repercussions to disclosing too much information as well. After growing up a poster child for childhood depression awareness and treatment, Claire went to work as a teacher, and found that parents and coworkers had a very different idea about how to talk to kids about mental health. At past teaching jobs, she has gotten in trouble with parents and administrators for being too candid about her own experience with depression, suicidal thoughts, and medication.

Alex had an even more harrowing experience. After quitting his medication in frustration a couple of years ago, he posted obliquely about his hopelessness on his Facebook wall. Someone he'd met through one of the social network's groups interpreted the post as a suicide threat and somehow notified the public safety department at Alex's college, which in turn sent the police to Alex's house. The police took him to the emergency room, where, although Alex insisted vehemently he wasn't suicidal, staff judged him a threat to himself and had him involuntarily committed to a psychiatric ward for two days. He considered the experience ironic, given his attempt to be hospitalized at the same unit four years earlier, when they told him they wouldn't admit him unless he had a plan to kill himself. The take-home lesson: he is far, far more careful about what he discloses, even to online "friends."

The issue of disclosure is far easier in any context, I think, if one can honestly say that one has been off medication for a long time and fared well ever since. Most people are primed to hear a version of the "overmedicated kid" or "angsty adolescent" narrative, and many agree with it. Even those who don't oppose medication for young people on principle usually want to think that problems are solvable, that as people mature they expand what one psychiatrist described to me as their "coping toolbox[es]." I hope this book will in some way enable my generation to speak more openly about this central, in many cases essential, part of their personal experience and life story.

Apart from fear of judgment and professional repercussions, discussing one's treatment in depth requires an assured and easily encapsulated attitude about medication that many people simply don't have. Not everyone who has spent years off meds is sure he will never relapse, or that she didn't sacrifice something in leaving the meds behind: greater productivity or focus, less anxiety and stress, better anger management. A lot of people think medication has been enormously helpful to them, yet express a vague desire to get off medication eventually, or to reduce their dosage, as though taking a lower dose were a sign of greater moral fortitude. Others are full of complaints about the drugs and the doctors who prescribed them, yet, with too many relapses under their belts, have resigned themselves to the prospect of taking drugs for life. And still others, myself included after researching this book, are curious to see how they might fare with fewer or no psychiatric drugs. Yet, to me at least, it never seems the right time to taper off. Life, and my own ambitions and self-expectations, not to mention my fear of relapse, keep getting in the way.

Even on a week-to-week or month-to-month basis, people's attitudes are remarkably volatile. You want to think that after so many years you know yourself and your symptoms well enough to have developed a coherent attitude toward your treatment. Yet one's experience of medication is so entwined in one's circumstances that whenever something changes—a new side effect appears, a relapse threatens, a relationship sours, a job dissolves—one is likely to wonder how well the drug is working, whether a switch or an augmentation is in order, or whether treatment is worth it after all.

Since my generation has grown up with so little guidance, discussion, or research about the short- and long-term effects of psychiatric medication, each individual is left to evaluate and interpret his or her own experiences. The constantly changing circumstances and shifting states of mind during young adulthood naturally influence our take on how medication is working in the present, but they also continue to inform our attempts to interpret and understand how medication has shaped us thus far and how it will affect us in the future. As T. S. Eliot put it, every new experience, every new moment brings "a hundred visions and revisions."

Our parents' generation was often not diagnosed until middle age; those whom the medications helped may have regretted that they hadn't received treatment earlier. In some cases they may even have been more willing to get their kids help at an earlier stage. Since many more people have now been medicated for psychiatric problems starting at a young age, the question arises: how will their experiences affect their approach to their children's treatment? Knowing that their kids are at an increased risk for inheriting their condition or a similar one, they will likely be more watchful for problems. In many cases, children will have inherited a similar psychic makeup—personality traits or tendencies that parents could interpret as precursors to later and more serious problems. Some evidence shows, not surprisingly, that parents who themselves had positive experiences with medication are more likely to endorse it for their children.[6] They might decide to wait and see, to intervene early, or, if their own experience with medication was roundly negative, to seek out different therapies or alternative treatments.

As time goes on, the number of young people who have grown up on medication increases. Unless new treatments or research cause a dramatic change in clinical practice, or a cultural backlash alters the current trends, this number is likely to grow apace, which makes it all the more important that we begin to discuss and study these medications' long-term physical and psychological effects. Some major longitudinal studies are in the works, and a small group of academics has begun to study children's subjective experiences with medications. Recently, a few widely publicized studies have questioned whether antidepressants are any more effective than placebos for mild to moderate depression, but the data is limited and the conclusions by no means definitive. Although the studies in question concern only antidepressants and their efficacy for very particular conditions, they have generated much discussion, playing as they do on society's understandable concern about widespread psychotropic medication use. Yet, as the placebo effect itself shows, what one expects of one's medication bears on its apparent effectiveness. Clearly, beliefs about meds are important, and it is urgent that we as a society also begin to discuss and to analyze the experiential components.

It is my hope that *Dosed* will encourage those who did grow up taking psychiatric drugs to share their ongoing experiences more openly. Then, those who care about us, those who are in a position to study and evaluate our experiences, and those who follow in our wake can better understand the true scope and impact of our society's psychotropic revolution.

Acknowledgments

I want first to thank my agent, Tracy Brown, who was responsible for getting this book off the ground and has been my great advocate along the way. I am deeply grateful to my editor at Beacon Press, Amy Caldwell, for believing in the importance of this topic, and for making me do this difficult but essential work of crafting and sustaining a compelling argument. Thank you as well to the publicity and marketing departments at Beacon, which have pushed this book enthusiastically from the get-go.

I'm indebted to the work of several social scientists whose research has shaped my thinking on the experience of taking medication from a young age. They include Eileen Anderson-Fye, Elizabeth Carpenter-Song, Jerry Floersch, David Karp, Jeffrey Longhofer, Tally Moses, and Ilina Singh. Also thanks to Richard A. Friedman at Weill Cornell Medical School, whose column in the *New York Times* planted the germ of an idea for this book.

I want to thank Glen Elliott and Gabrielle Carlson for their patient and helpful overviews of the historical changes in child psychiatry research over recent decades, and Julie Magno Zito, whose research has been an invaluable source of statistics and who provided an incisive summary of the state of epidemiological research regarding children and psychotropics. A number of clinicians generously shared their clinical experiences and professional observations, including Sharon Bisco, Debra Emmite, Sherry Goldman, Kevin Kalikow, David Mintz, Kevin Passer, John Scialli, and Steven Warres. Laurel Leslie helped me get acquainted with the workings of foster-care systems. Nina Burleigh at Columbia University School of Journalism provided my earliest guidance and encouragement in pursuing this topic, first for a graduate seminar, and then as a book. Steve Tannenbaum was my perceptive and thoughtful correspondent, exploring and expounding upon this book's themes. And Carla Massey has been a continual source of information, advice, and support since before this project began.

Thanks also to everyone who made it possible for me to travel around the country to interview and visit the five young people I follow closely in this book. And thank you, of course, to the many "grown-up medicated kids" whom I interviewed for this book—most especially, of course, Alex, Caleb, Claire, Elizabeth, and Paul, who gave so generously of their time and shared so many of their experiences and thoughts with me.

My sister, Amanda, has offered a sounding board and a sympathetic ear and has been my unwavering cheerleader. My father helped get this project going by insisting, with his infinite enthusiasm and faith in my abilities, that I could indeed write a book, and has remained, as always, my unflagging booster. And the deepest thanks to my mother, who invested a great deal in the writing process, gamely brainstorming with me when I got stuck and providing truly invaluable comments, suggestions, and edits. Finally, thanks to my husband, Michael, who endured my often single-minded devotion to this book for the duration of our engagement and our first year of marriage. He pushes me to aim even higher than I would aim myself, and will always be a fellow journalist in my mind.

Notes

INTRODUCTION

1. Peter D. Kramer, *Listening to Prozac*, 2nd ed. (New York: Penguin Books, 1997), 221.
2. Tally Moses and Stuart A. Kirk, "Psychosocial Side Effects of Drug Treatment of Youth," in *Mental Disorders in the Social Environment: Critical Perspectives*, ed. Stuart A. Kirk (New York: Columbia University Press, 2005), 389.
3. Richard A. Friedman, "Who Are We? Coming of Age on Antidepressants," *New York Times*, April 15, 2008.
4. Andrew Solomon, *The Noonday Demon* (New York: Scribner, 2001), 15.
5. David Healy, *Let Them Eat Prozac: The Unhealthy Relationship between the Pharmaceutical Industry and Depression* (New York: New York University Press, 2004), 9, 35.
6. Julie Magno Zito, Daniel J. Safer, Susan dosReis, et al., "Psychotropic Practice Patterns for Youth: A 10-Year Perspective," *Archives of Pediatrics and Adolescent Medicine* 157 (January 2003): 17–25; Mark Olfson, Steven C. Marcus, Myrna Weissman, and Peter S. Jensen, "National Trends in the Use of Psychotropic Medications by Children," *Journal of the American Academy of Child and Adolescent Psychiatry* 41, no. 5 (2002): 514–21.
7. Cindy Parks Thomas, Peter Conrad, Rosemary Casler, and Elizabeth Goodman, "Trends in the Use of Psychotropic Medications among Adolescents, 1994 to 2001," *Psychiatric Services* 57, no. 1 (January 2006): 64.

8. Robert P. Gallagher, *National Survey of Counseling Center Directors, 2009*, Monograph Series Number 8R (Alexandria, VA: International Association of Counseling Services), 6.

9. Benedetto Vitiello, "Pharmacoepidemiology and Pediatric Psychopharmacology Research," *Journal of Child and Adolescent Psychopharmacology* 15, no. 1 (2005): 10–11.

10. Data Resource Center for Child and Adolescent Health, "2007 National Survey of Children's Health," http://childhealthdata.org.

11. Renee Goodwin, Madelyn S. Gould, Carlos Blanco, and Mark Olfson, "Prescription of Psychotropic Medications to Youths in Office-Based Practice," *Psychiatric Services* 52, no. 8 (August 2001): 1081.

12. Mark A. Riddle, Elizabeth A. Kastelic, and Emily Frosch, "Pediatric Psychopharmacology," *Journal of Child Psychology and Psychiatry* 42, no. 1 (2001): 74.

13. Benedetto Vitiello, "Recent NIMH Clinical Trials and Implications for Practice," *Journal of the American Academy of Child and Adolescent Psychiatry* 47, no. 12 (December 2008): 1369–74; TADS Team, "The Treatment for Adolescents with Depression Study (TADS): Long-term Effectiveness and Safety Outcomes," *Archives of General Psychiatry* 64, no. 10 (October 2007): 1132–44.

14. Erik Parens and Josephine Johnston, "Facts, Values and Attention-Deficit Hyperactivity Disorder (ADHD): Update on the Controversies," *Child and Adolescent Psychiatry and Mental Health* 3, no. 1 (January 2009).

15. Marcia Angell, "The Epidemic of Mental Illness: Why?" *New York Review of Books*, June 23, 2011, 20–22.

16. Peter Kramer, "In Defense of Antidepressants," *New York Times*, July 9, 2011.

17. For an in-depth examination, see Robert Whitaker, *Anatomy of an Epidemic* (New York: Crown, 2010).

CHAPTER I: DIFFICULT KIDS

1. Jonathan Metzl, *Prozac on the Couch: Prescribing Gender in the Era of Wonder Drugs* (Durham, NC: Duke University Press, 2003), Google e-book, section 51; Alan E. Kazdin, "Child and Adolescent Psychotherapy," in *Encyclopedia of Psychology*, vol. 2 (Washington, DC: American Psychological Association, 2000).

2. Alan E. Kazdin, "Behavior Therapy," in *Encyclopedia of Psychology*, vol. 2 (Washington, DC: American Psychological Association, 2000).

3. Leon Eisenberg, "Mindlessness and Brainlessness in Psychiatry," *British Journal of Psychiatry* 148 (May 1986): 497–508.

4. Marcia Angell, "The Illusions of Psychiatry," *New York Review of Books*, July 14, 2011.

5. Mina K. Dulcan, *Dulcan's Textbook of Child and Adolescent Psychiatry*, part 881 (Arlington, VA: American Psychiatric Publishing, 2010), 63.

6. Ronald C. Kessler, Patricia Berglund, Olga Demler, et al., "Lifetime Prevalence and Age-of-Onset distributions of DSM-IV Disorders in the National Co-morbidity Survey Replication," *Archives of General Psychiatry* 62, no. 6 (2005): 593–602.

7. Stanley Greenspan, *The Challenging Child* (Reading, MA: Addison-Wesley, 1995).

8. Zito et al., "Rising Prevalence of Antidepressants."

9. "Antidepressants Called Rising Risk for Children," *Associated Press* report, *New York Times*, November 23, 1980.

10. Riddle, Kastelic, and Frosch, "Pediatric Psychopharmacology," 81, 89.

11. Frederick J. Frese III, "The Mental Health Service Consumer's Perspective on Mandatory Treatment," *New Directions for Mental Health Services* 75 (1997): 17.

12. David G. Fassler and Lynne S. Dumas, *Help Me, I'm Sad: Recognizing, Treating, and Preventing Childhood and Adolescent Depression* (New York: Penguin, 1997), 76.

13. Lawrence Diller, "The Run on Ritalin: Attention Deficit Disorder and Stimulant Treatment in the 1990s," *Hastings Center Report* 26, no. 2 (March–April 1996): 12.

14. Andrew Purvis and Philip Elmer-DeWitt, "Why Junior Won't Sit Still," *Time*, November 29, 1990.

15. Daniel J. Safer, Julie M. Zito, and Eric M. Fine, "Increased Methylphenidate Usage for Attention Deficit Disorder in the 1990s," *Pediatrics* 98, no. 6 (1996): 1084–88.

16. Alvin A. Rosenfeld et al., "Foster Care Children—An Update Journal," *Journal of the American Academy of Child and Adolescent Psychiatry* 36, no. 4 (1997): 454.

17. Susan dosReis et al., "Mental Health Services for Youth in Foster Care and Disabled Youth," *American Journal of Public Health* 91, no. 7 (July 2001): 1094.

18. Christopher R. Thomas and Charles E. Holzer, "National Distribution of Child and Adolescent Psychiatrists," *Journal of the American Academy of Child and Adolescent Psychiatry* 38, no. 1 (January 1999): 9–15.

19. Zito et al., "Rising Prevalence of Antidepressants," 723.

20. Ibid., 724.

21. Amanda J. Hirsch and John S. Carlson, "Prescription Practices and Empirical Efficacy of Psychopharmacologic Treatments for Pediatric Major Depressive Disorder," *Journal of Child and Adolescent Psychiatric Nursing* 20, no. 4 (2007): 228.

CHAPTER 2: PLAYING A ROLE

1. Kramer, *Listening to Prozac*, 41, 146–49.

2. Mary Lou de Leon Siantz, "The Stigma of Mental Illness on Children of Color," *Journal of Child and Adolescent Psychiatric Nursing* 6, no. 4 (1993): 13.

3. Jeffrey Longhofer and Jerry Floersch, "Desire and Disappointment: Adolescent Psychotropic Treatment and Adherence," *Anthropology & Medicine* 17, no. 2 (August 2010): 159–72.

4. Tally Moses, "Adolescents' Commitment to Continuing Psychotropic Medication: A Preliminary Investigation of Considerations, Contradictions, and Correlates," *Child Psychiatry and Human Development* 42 (2011): 108.

5. Vanya Hamrin, Erin M. McCarthy, and Veda Tyson, "Pediatric Psychotropic Medication Initiation and Adherence: A Literature Review Based on Social Exchange Theory," *Journal of Child and Adolescent Psychiatric Nursing* 23, no. 3 (August 2010): 151.

6. Edward M. Hallowell and John J. Ratey, *Driven to Distraction: Recognizing and Coping with Attention Deficit Disorder from Childhood through Adulthood* (New York: Pantheon Books, 1994), 52, 152.

7. Olfson et al., "National Trends in the Use of Psychotropic Medications by Children," 518.

8. Jonathan S. Comer, Mark Olfson, and Ramin Mojtabai, "National Trends in Child and Adolescent Psychotropic Polypharmacy in Office-Based Practice, 1996–2007," *Journal of the American Academy of Child and Adolescent Psychiatry* 49, no. 10 (October 2010): 1001–10.

9. Daniel J. Safer, Julie Magno Zito, and Susan dosReis, "Concomitant Psychotropic Medication for Youths," *American Journal of Psychiatry* 160, no. 3 (2003): 440.

10. Goodwin et al., "Prescription of Psychotropic Medications to Youths in Office-Based Practice," 1085.

11. Ramin Mojtabai and Mark Olfson, "National Trends in Psychotherapy by Office-Based Psychiatrists," *Archives of General Psychiatry* 68, no. 8 (2008): 964.

12. Mark Olfson, Steven C. Marcus, Benjamin Druss, and Harold Alan Pincus, "National Trends in the Use of Outpatient Psychotherapy," *American Journal of Psychiatry* 159, no. 11 (November 2002): 1914.

13. Patrick E. Jamieson, *Mind Race* (Oxford, UK: Oxford University Press, 2006), 21.

14. Janice Martin, "Bringing Order to Disorder," *St. Petersburg (Florida) Times*, August 5, 1990.

15. Esther K. Sleator, Rina K. Ullmann, and Alice von Neumann, "How Do Hyperactive Children Feel about Taking Stimulants, and Will They Tell the Doctor?" *Clinical Pediatrics* 21 (1982): 474, 479.

16. Carol K. Whalen, "Attention Deficit and Hyperactivity Disorders," in *Handbook of Child Psychopathology*, eds. Thomas H. Ollendick and Michael Hersen (New York: Plenum, 1983), 187.

17. Diller, "The Run on Ritalin," 16.

18. Enid M. Hunkeler et al., "Trends in the Use of Antidepressants, Lithium and Anticonvulsants in Kaiser Permanente-Insured Youths, 1994–2003," *Journal of Child and Adolescent Psychopharmacology* 15, no. 1 (2005): 26–37; Julie Magno Zito, Daniel J. Safer, James F. Gardner, et al., "Anticonvulsant Treatment for Psychiatric and Seizure Indication among Youths," *Psychiatric Services* 57 (2006): 681–85; Goodwin et al., "Prescription of Psychotropic Medications to Youths in Office-Based Practice," 1085.

CHAPTER 3: SCHOOL INTERVENTIONS

1. Ilina Singh, "Not Just Naughty: 50 Years of Stimulant Drug Advertising," in *Medicating Modern America: Prescriptions Drugs in History*, eds. Andrea Tone and Elizabeth Siegel Watkins (New York: New York University Press, 2007), 147.

2. Daniel J. Safer and John M. Krager, "Effect of a Media Blitz and a Threatened Lawsuit on Stimulant Treatment," *Journal of the American Medical Association* 268, no. 8 (August 26, 1992): 1004, 1007; Lee Mitgang, " 'R' is for Ritalin," *Associated Press*, April 6, 1988; Diane Divoky, "Ritalin: Education's Fix-It Drug?" *Phi Delta Kappan* 70, no. 8 (April 1989): 600.

3. Judith Warner, *We've Got Issues: Children and Parents in the Age of Medication* (New York: Riverhead Books, 2010), 104–6.

4. Susan D. Mayes, Susan L. Calhoun, and Errin W. Crowell, "Learning Disabilities and ADHD: Overlapping Spectrum Disorders," *Journal of Learning Disabilities* 33, no. 5 (2000): 417–24; Russell A. Barkley, "What to Look for in a School for a Child with ADHD," *ADHD Report* 2, no. 3 (1994): 1–3.

5. Sally Reed, "Whatever Happened to Alternative Schools?" *New York Times*, November 15, 1981.

6. Michael A. W. Ottey, "Second-Chance Schools Grow Despite Few Success Stories," *Oregonian*, June 26, 2000.

7. Steven Mintz, *Huck's Raft: A History of American Childhood* (Cambridge, MA: Harvard University Press), 369–70.

8. Robert E. McGrath, "Prescriptive Authority for Psychologists," *Annual Review of Clinical Psychology* 6 (April 2010): 29.

9. Ruth Shalit, "Defining Disability Down," *New Republic*, August 27, 1997, 16–22; Susan M. Vess, "Americans with Disabilities Act," in *Encyclopedia of School Psychology*, ed. Steven W. Lee (Thousand Oaks, CA: Sage, 2005), 22–23.

10. Lawrence H. Diller, "The Last Normal Child: America's Intolerance of Di-

versity in Children's Performance and Behavior," in *The Last Normal Child*, ed. Lawrence H. Diller (Westport, CT: Greenwood, 2006), 42.

11. Abigail Sullivan Moore, "Accommodations Angst," *New York Times*, November 4, 2010.

12. William E. Pelham Jr., Betsy Hoza, Heidi L. Kipp, et al., "Effects of Methylphenidate and Expectancy on ADHD Children's Performance, Self-Evaluations, Persistence, and Attributions on a Cognitive Task," *Experimental and Clinical Psychopharmacology* 5, no. 1 (1997): 1–13.

13. Mona M. Shattell, Robin Bartlett, and Tracie Rowe, "'I Have Always Felt Different': The Experience of Attention-Deficit/Hyperactivity Disorder in Childhood," *Journal of Pediatric Nursing* 23, no. 1 (February 2008): 52.

14. John McGinnis, "Attention Deficit Disaster," *Wall Street Journal*, September 18, 1997.

CHAPTER 4: EARLY REBELLIONS

1. Sabine Hack and Byron Chow, "Pediatric Psychotropic Medication Compliance: A Literature Review and Research-Based Suggestions for Improving Treatment Compliance," *Journal of Child and Adolescent Psychopharmacology* 11, no. 1 (2001): 61.

2. Alice Charach, "Understanding Treatment Adherence in Children with Attention-Deficit/Hyperactivity Disorder," *Psychiatric Times*, October 1, 2008.

3. Jeffrey Longhofer, Jerry Floersch, and Nate Okpych, "Foster Youth and Psychotropic Treatment: Where Next?" *Children and Youth Services Review* 33, no. 2 (February 2011): 400.

4. David A. Karp, *Is It Me or My Meds? Living with Antidepressants* (Cambridge, MA: Harvard University Press, 2006), 166–67.

5. Jerry Floersch, "The Subjective Experience of Youth Psychotropic Treatment," *Social Work in Mental Health* 1, no. 4 (2003): 57–58.

6. Jon McClellan and John Werry, "Practice Parameters for the Assessment and Treatment of Children and Adolescents with Bipolar Disorder," *Journal of the American Academy of Child and Adolescent Psychiatry* 36, no. 1 (January 1997): 140.

7. Mark Olfson, Carlos Blanc, Linxu Liu, et al., "National Trends in the Outpatient Treatment of Children and Adolescents with Antipsychotic Drugs," *Archives of General Psychiatry* 63 (2006): 679–85.

8. McClellan and Werry, "Practice Parameters for the Assessment and Treatment of Children and Adolescents with Bipolar Disorder," 140.

9. For a summary of studies, see Allison M. R. Lee and Igor I. Galynker, "Violence in Bipolar Disorder: What Role Does Trauma Play?" *Psychiatric Times*, November 17, 2010.

10. For a summary of findings, see Julie M. Zito, Daniel J. Safer, Devadatta Sai, et al., "Psychotropic Medication Patterns among Youth in Foster Care," *Pediatrics* 121, no. 1 (January 2008): e158; Bonnie T. Zima, Regina Bussing, Gia M. Crecelius, et al., "Psychotropic Medication Use among Children in Foster Care: Relationship to Severe Psychiatric Disorders," *American Journal of Public Health* 89, no. 11 (November 1999): 1732–35.

11. Zito et al., "Psychotropic Medication Patterns," e161.

12. For a summary of the literature, see Moses, "Adolescents' Commitment to Continuing Psychotropic Medication," 94.

13. Ibid., 95; Hamrin, McCarthy, and Tyson, "Pediatric Psychotropic Medication Initiation and Adherence," 162; Catherine Laurier, Denis Lafortune, and Johanne Collin, "Compliance with Psychotropic Medication Treatment among Adolescents Living in Youth Care Centres," *Children and Youth Services Review* 32 (2010): 72.

14. Moses and Kirk, "Psychosocial Side Effects," 398.

15. Jennifer Egan, "The Thin Red Line," *New York Times Magazine*, July 27, 1997.

16. Peter D. Kramer, *Against Depression* (New York: Penguin Books, 2005), 213–14, 224.

17. Elizabeth Wurtzel, *Prozac Nation: Young and Depressed in America* (Boston: Houghton Mifflin, 1994), 289.

18. Hack and Chow, "Pediatric Psychotropic Medication Compliance," 63–64.

19. Hamrin, McCarthy, and Tyson, "Pediatric Psychotropic Medication Initiation and Adherence," 161.

20. Moses, "Adolescents' Commitment to Continuing Psychotropic Medication," 95; Hamrin, McCarthy, and Tyson, "Pediatric Psychotropic Medication Initiation and Adherence," 160; Hack and Chow, "Pediatric Psychotropic Medication Compliance," 63–64.

21. Eileen Anderson-Fye, co-principal investigator of Case Western Reserve University Presidential Research Initiative Grant, "College Student Experience of Mental Health Service Use and Psychiatric Medication," interview with the author, July 2011.

22. Moses, "Adolescents' Commitment to Continuing Psychotropic Medication," 107.

23. United Press International, "New Drug Treats Kids' Compulsions," March 26, 1997.

24. Fassler and Dumas, *Help Me, I'm Sad*, 143.

25. "Practice Parameters for the Assessment and Treatment of Children and Adolescents with Obsessive-Compulsive Disorder," *Journal of the American Academy of Child and Adolescent Psychiatry* 37, no. 10 supplement (1998): 41S, 38S.

CHAPTER 5: SOMETHING NEW?

1. Colette Dowling, "Rescuing Your Child from Depression," *New York Magazine*, January 20, 1992, 46.

2. Robert M. Post and Susan R. B. Weiss, "Sensitization and Kindling Phenomena in Mood, Anxiety, and Obsessive-Compulsive Disorders: The Role of Serotonergic Mechanisms in Illness Progression," *Biological Psychiatry* 44, no. 3 (August 1998): 193–206.

3. Amy Cheung, Vivek Kusumakar, Stan Kutcher, et al., "Maintenance Study for Adolescent Depression," *Journal of Child and Adolescent Psychopharmacology* 18, no. 4 (August 2008): 389.

4. Edmund S. Higgins, "Do ADHD Drugs Take a Toll on the Brain?" *Scientific American Mind*, July–August 2009; Ekaterina Staikova, David J. Marks, Carlin J. Miller, et al., "Childhood Stimulant Treatment and Teen Depression: Is There a Relationship?" *Journal of Child and Adolescent Psychopharmacology* 20, no. 5 (October 2010): 387.

5. McClellan and Werry, "Practice Parameters for the Assessment and Treatment of Children and Adolescents with Bipolar Disorder," 139.

6. Michael Strober and Gabrielle Carlson, "Bipolar Illness in Adolescents with Major Depression: Clinical, Genetic, and Psychopharmacologic Predictors in a Three- to Four-Year Prospective Follow-up Investigation," *Archives of General Psychiatry* 39, no. 10 (May 1982): 555.

7. Kiki D. Chang, Kirti Saxena, et al., "Psychotropic Medication Exposure and Age at Onset of Bipolar Disorder in Offspring of Parents with Bipolar Disorder," *Journal of Child and Adolescent Psychopharmacology* 20, no. 1 (2010): 25.

8. Whitaker, *Anatomy of an Epidemic*, 190–226.

9. Chang et al., "Psychotropic Medication Exposure and Age at Onset of Bipolar Disorder in Offspring of Parents with Bipolar Disorder," 29–30.

10. Andres Martin, Christopher Young, James F. Leckman, et al., "Age Effects on Antidepressant-Induced Manic Conversion," *Archives of Pediatric and Adolescent Medicine* 158 (August 2004): 776, 777.

CHAPTER 6: BREAKDOWNS

1. Solomon, *The Noonday Demon*, 81.

2. Frank Owen, "The Brooklyn Girls Fight Club," *Maxim*, June 9, 2008.

3. Kay Redfield Jamison, *An Unquiet Mind* (New York: Random House Digital, 1996), Google e-book, 110.

4. Ibid., 115.

5. Frederick J. Frese and Wendy Walker Davis, "The Consumer-Survivor Movement, Recovery, and Consumer Professionals," *Professional Psychology: Research and Practice* 28, no. 3 (1997): 244.

6. Jeffrey L. Geller and Kathleen Biebel, "The Premature Demise of Public Child and Adolescent Inpatient Psychiatric Beds," *Psychiatric Quarterly* 77 (2006): 255.

7. Ibid.; Robert M. Friedman and Krista Kutash, "Challenges for Child and Adolescent Mental Health," *Health Affairs* (Fall 1992): 129.

8. Warner, *We've Got Issues*, 47.

9. Geller and Biebel, "The Premature Demise," 255–56.

10. Government Accountability Office, *Young Adults with Serious Mental Illness*, GAO Report 08-678 (Washington, DC: June 2008), 3–4.

11. Martha Anne Kitzrow, "The Mental Health Needs of Today's College Students: Challenges and Recommendations," *NASPA Journal* 41, no. 1 (Fall 2003): 167.

12. Rebecca Trounson, "Report Faults UC's Mental Health Care," *Los Angeles Times*, September 20, 2006, 4.

13. Richard Kadison and Theresa Foy DiGeronimo, *College of the Overwhelmed: The Campus Mental Health Crisis and What to Do about It* (San Francisco: Jossey-Bass, 2004).

14. Ibid., 91.

CHAPTER 7: SIDE EFFECTS

1. Wurtzel, *Prozac Nation*, 1, 2.

2. Ibid., 2, 4, 16, 17.

3. Moses and Kirk, "Psychosocial Side Effects," 388–89; Jennifer Bowen, Terence Fenton, and Leonard Rappaport, "Stimulant Treatment and Attention-Deficit Hyperactivity Disorder: The Child's Perspective," *American Journal of Diseases of Children* 145 (1991): 291–95.

4. Elyn R. Saks, *The Center Cannot Hold* (New York: Hyperion, 2007), 264.

5. "The Carlat Quick Guide to Atypical Antipsychotics," *Carlat Psychiatry Report* 9, no. 6 (June 2011).

6. Alex Berenson, "Lilly to Pay $690 Million in Drug Suits," *New York Times*, June 10, 2005.

7. Benedict Carey, "Risks Found for Youths in New Antipsychotics," *New York Times*, September 15, 2008; Gardiner Harris, "Use of Antipsychotics in Children Is Criticized," *New York Times*, November 18, 2008.

8. Angell, "The Illusions of Psychiatry."

9. Duff Wilson, "For $520 Million, Astro-Zeneca Settles Case over Marketing of a Drug," *New York Times*, April 28, 2010.

10. Alexander M. Scharko, "Selective Serotonin Reuptake Inhibitor–Induced Sexual Dysfunction in Adolescents: A Review," *Journal of the American Academy of Child and Adolescent Psychiatry* 43, no. 9 (September 2004): 1076.

11. Ibid.

12. John Walkup and Michael Labellarte, "Complications of SSRI Treatment," *Journal of Child and Adolescent Psychopharmacology* 11, no. 1 (2001): 1.

13. "Teen Pregnancy: Trends and Lessons Learned," *Guttmacher Report on Public Policy* 5, no. 1 (February 2002): 7–8; Mintz, *Huck's Raft*, 336, 346, 361–62.

14. M. C. Shearer and S. L. Bermingham, "The Ethics of Paediatric Antidepressant Use: Erring on the Side of Caution," *Journal of Medication Ethics* 34, no. 10 (October 2008): 711.

15. Michael E. Thase, Harald Murck, and Anke Post, "Clinical Relevance of Disturbances of Sleep and Vigilance in Major Depressive Disorder: A Review," *Primary Care Companion to the Journal of Clinical Psychiatry* 12, no. 6 (2010): e1–e10.

16. Raul R. Silva, Jeffrey W. Skimming, and Rafael Muniz, "Cardiovascular Safety of Stimulant Medications for Pediatric Attention-Deficit Hyperactivity Disorder," *Clinical Pediatrics* 49, no. 9 (2010): 846.

CHAPTER 8: COMPLICATING FACTORS

1. H. Steven Moffic, "The Meaning of Life in a 15-Minute Med Check, *Couch in Crisis* [blog], *Psychiatric Times*, May 19, 2011.

2. Jack Drescher, "A History of Homosexuality and Organized Psychoanalysis," *Journal of the American Academy of Psychoanalysis and Dynamic Psychiatry* 36, no. 3 (Fall 2008): 446, 447.

3. Ritch C. Savin-Williams, *The New Gay Teenager* (Cambridge, MA: Harvard University Press, 2005), Google e-book, 72.

4. Drescher, "A History of Homosexuality," 450.

5. Metzl, *Prozac on the Couch*, 31.

6. Miriam Rosenberg, "Recognizing Gay, Lesbian, and Transgender Teens in a Child and Adolescent Psychiatry Practice," *Journal of the American Academy of Child and Adolescent Psychiatry* 42, no. 12 (December 2003): 1517–18.

7. Savin-Williams, *The New Gay Teenager*, 50.

8. Substance Abuse and Mental Health Services Administration, *Results from the 2009 National Survey on Drug Use and Health*, vol. 1, *Summary of National Findings*, NSDUH Series H-38A, HHS Publication no. SMA 10-4586 Findings (Rockville, MD: Office of Applied Studies, 2010), 31.

9. Daniel Carlat, "A Primer on Drug Testing," *Carlat Psychiatry Report* 8, no. 5 (May 2010): 3.

10. James M. Bolton, Jennifer Robinson, and Jitender Sareen, "Self-Medication of Mood Disorders with Alcohol and Drugs in the National Epidemiologic Survey on Alcohol and Related Conditions," *Journal of Affective Disorders* 115, no. 3 (June 2009): 367–75.

11. Jeffrey Jensen Arnett, "The Developmental Context of Substance Use in Emerging Adulthood," *Journal of Drug Issues* (2005): 240.

12. Russell A. Barkley, Mariellen Fischer, et al., "Does the Treatment of Attention-Deficit/Hyperactivity Disorder with Stimulants Contribute to Drug Use/Abuse? A 13-Year Prospective Study," *Pediatrics* 111, no. 1 (January 2003): 97.

13. See Higgins, "Do ADHD Drugs Take a Toll on the Brain?"

14. Carlat, "A Primer on Drug Testing," 3.

15. Substance Abuse and Mental Health Services Administration, *Results from the 2009 National Survey on Drug Use and Health*, 19–20.

16. Robert J. Fortuna, Brett W. Robbins, and Enrico Caiola, "Prescribing of Controlled Medications to Adolescents and Young Adults in the United States," *Pediatrics* 126, no. 6 (December 2010), 1114.

17. Abigail Ortiz, Pablo Cervantes, Gregorio Zlotnik, et al., "Cross-prevalence of Migraine and Bipolar Disorder, *Bipolar Disorders* 12, no. 4 (June 2006): 397–403; American Headache Society, "The American Migraine Prevalence and Prevention Study Fact Sheet," http://www.headaches.org.

18. T. W. Victor, X. Hu, and J. C. Campbell, "Migraine Prevalence by Age and Sex in the United States: A Life-Span Study," *Cephalalgia: An International Journal of Headache* 30, no. 9 (September 2010): 1065–72; Fred D. Sheftell and Marcelo E. Bigal, "Headache and Psychiatric Comorbidity," *Psychiatric Times*, November 1, 2004.

19. Karp, *Is It Me or My Meds?* 57.

20. Deborah R. Kim, L. Gyulai, and E. W. Freeman, "Premenstrual Dysphoric Disorder and Psychiatric Co-morbidity," *Archives of Women's Mental Health* 7 (2004): 41–43.

21. Alan F. Schatzburg, Jonathan O. Cole, and Charles DeBattista, *Manual of Clinical Psychopharmacology* (Arlington, VA: American Psychiatric Publishing, 2010), 596; Donna E. Stewart and Gail Erlick Robinson, "Psychotropic Drugs and Electroconvulsive Therapy in Pregnancy and Lactation," in *Psychological Aspects of Women's Health Care*, eds. Nada Logan Stotland and Donna E. Stewart (Arlington, VA: American Psychiatric Publishing, 2001), 69.

22. The American College of Obstetricians and Gynecologists, "Use of Psychiatric Medications during Pregnancy and Lactation," *Obstetrics and Gynecology* 111, no. 4 (April 2008): 1002–4.

23. Adele C. Viguera, Theodore Whitfield, Ross Baldessarini, et al., "Risk of Recurrence in Women with Bipolar Disorder during Pregnancy: Prospective Study of Mood Stabilizer Discontinuation," *American Journal of Psychiatry* 164, no. 12 (December 2007): 1817–24; Lee S. Cohen, Lori L. Altshuler, Bernard L. Harlow, et al., "Relapse of Major Depression during Pregnancy in Women Who Maintain or Discontinue Antidepressant Treatment," *Journal of the American Medical Association* 295, no. 5 (February 2006): 499–507.

24. Talia Puzantian, "Psychotropics in Pregnancy and Breastfeeding: A Comprehensive Chart," *Carlat Psychiatry Report* 8, no. 11 (November 2010): 3.

25. Deanna Nobleza, "Antidepressant Treatment in Pregnancy: An Update," *Carlat Psychiatry Report* 8, no. 11 (November 2010): 4.
26. Kimberly A. Yonkers, Katherine L. Wisner, Donna E. Stewart, et al., "The Management of Depression during Pregnancy: A Report from the American Psychiatric Association and the American College of Obstetricians and Gynecologists," *Obstetrics and Gynecology* 114, no. 3 (September 2009): 703–13.
27. Mayo Clinic, "Antidepressants: Safe during Pregnancy?" http://www.mayo clinic.com.
28. Cohen, Altshuler, Harlow, et al., "Relapse of Major Depression during Pregnancy," 130.
29. British Psychological Society and Royal College of Psychiatrists, "The Pharmacological Treatment of Mental Disorders in Pregnant and Breastfeeding Women," in *Antenatal and Postnatal Mental Health* (Leicester, UK: National Collaborating Center for Mental Health, 2007), 201; MGH Center for Women's Mental Health, "Anxiety during Pregnancy: How Does It Affect the Developing Fetal Brain?" April 11, 2011, http://www.womensmental health.org.

CHAPTER 9: REASSESSMENTS

1. Kevin M. McKay, Zac E. Imel, and Bruce E. Wampold, "Psychiatrist Effects in the Pharmacological Treatment of Depression," *Journal of Affective Disorders* 92, nos. 2–3 (June 2006): 287–90; Eilis Kennedy, "Evaluating Interventions in Child Mental Health: The Importance of Care Provider and Contextual Influences," *Clinical Child Psychology and Psychiatry* 14, no. 2 (2009): 163–65.
2. Kathleen J. Pottick, Scott Bilder, Ann Vander Stoep, et al., "U.S. Patterns of Mental Health Service Utilization for Transition-Age Youth and Young Adults," *Journal of Behavioral Health Services & Research* 35, no. 4 (October 2008): 381, 382.
3. Carmen DeNavas-Walt, Bernadette D. Proctor, and Jessica C. Smith, *U.S. Census Bureau, Current Population Reports, P60-239, Income, Poverty, and Health Insurance Coverage in the United States: 2010* (Washington, DC: U.S. Government Printing Office, 2011), 26; Karen Schwartz and Tanya Schwartz, *Uninsured Young Adults: A Profile and Overview of Coverage Options* (Washington, DC: Kaiser Commission Medicaid and the Uninsured, 2008), 1–3.
4. Samantha A. Stewart, "Effects of Benzodiazepines on Cognition," *Journal of Clinical Psychiatry* 66, supplement 2 (2005): 9.
5. Lauren Slater, *Prozac Diary* (New York: Penguin Books, 1999), 116.
6. Hamrin, McCarthy, and Tyson, "Pediatric Psychotropic Medication Initiation and Adherence," 160.